Also Available From the American Academy of Pediatrics

Common Conditions

Allergies and Asthma: What Every Parent Needs to Know

The Big Book of Symptoms: A–Z Guide to Your Child's Health

Mama Doc Medicine: Finding Calm and Confidence in Parenting, Child Health, and Work-Life Balance

My Child Is Sick! Expert Advice for Managing Common Illnesses and Injuries

Sleep: What Every Parent Needs to Know

Waking Up Dry: A Guide to Help Children Overcome Bedwetting

Developmental, Behavioral, and Psychosocial Information

ADHD: What Every Parent Needs to Know

Autism Spectrum Disorders: What Every Parent Needs to Know

CyberSafe: Protecting and Empowering Kids in the Digital World of Texting, Gaming, and Social Media

Mental Health, Naturally: The Family Guide to Holistic Care for a Healthy Mind and Body

Newborns, Infants, and Toddlers

Baby Care Anywhere: A Quick Guide to Parenting On the Go

Caring for Your Baby and Young Child: Birth to Age 5*

Dad to Dad: Parenting Like a Pro

Guide to Toilet Training*

Heading Home With Your Newborn: From Birth to Reality

Mommy Calls: Dr. Tanya Answers Parents' Top 101 Questions About Babies and Toddlers

New Mother's Guide to Breastfeeding*

Raising Twins: Parenting Multiples From Pregnancy Through the School Years

Retro Baby: Cut Back on All the Gear and Boost Your Baby's Development With More Than 100 Time-tested Activities

Understanding the NICU: What Parents of Preemies and Other Hospitalized Newborns Need to Know

Your Baby's First Year*

Nutrition and Fitness

Food Fights: Winning the Nutritional Challenges of Parenthood Armed With Insight, Humor, and a Bottle of Ketchup

Nutrition: What Every Parent Needs to Know

A Parent's Guide to Childhood Obesity: A Road Map to Health

Sports Success Rx! Your Child's Prescription for the Best Experience

School-aged Children and Adolescents

Building Resilience in Children and Teens: Giving Kids Roots and Wings

Raising Kids to Thrive: Balancing Love With Expectations and Protection With Trust

For additional parenting resources, visit the HealthyChildren bookstore at

shop.aap.org/for-parents.

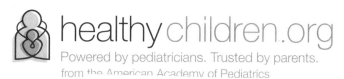

The Picky Eater Project

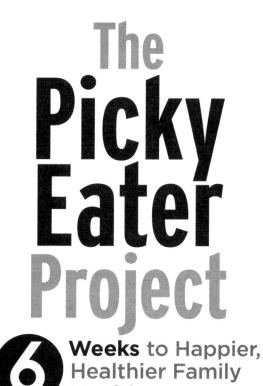

6 **Weeks** to Happier, Healthier Family Mealtimes

Natalie Digate Muth, MD, MPH, RDN, FAAP

AND

Sally Sampson, Founder, ChopChop Kids

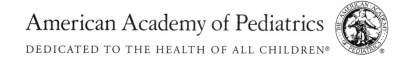

American Academy of Pediatrics

DEDICATED TO THE HEALTH OF ALL CHILDREN®

American Academy of Pediatrics Publishing Staff

Mark Grimes, *Director, Department of Publishing*

Kathryn Sparks, *Manager, Consumer Publishing*

Holly Kaminski, *Editor, Consumer Publishing*

Shannan Martin, *Production Manager, Consumer Publications*

Amanda Helmholz, *Editorial Specialist*

Linda Diamond, *Manager, Art Direction and Production*

Mary Lou White, *Director, Department of Marketing and Sales*

Sara Hoerdeman, *Marketing Manager, Consumer Products*

About the American Academy of Pediatrics

The American Academy of Pediatrics is an organization of 66,000 primary care pediatricians, pediatric medical subspecialists, and pediatric surgical specialists dedicated to the health, safety, and well-being of infants, children, adolescents, and young adults.

Published by the American Academy of Pediatrics
141 Northwest Point Blvd
Elk Grove Village, IL 60007-1019
Telephone: 847/434-4000
Facsimile: 847/434-8000
www.aap.org

The information contained in this publication should not be used as a substitute for the medical care and advice of your pediatrician. There may be variations in treatment that your pediatrician may recommend based on individual facts and circumstances.

Statements and opinions expressed are those of the authors and not necessarily those of the American Academy of Pediatrics.

Listing of resources does not imply an endorsement by the American Academy of Pediatrics (AAP). The AAP is not responsible for the content of external resources. Information was current at the time of publication.

Products and Web sites are mentioned for informational purposes only and do not imply an endorsement by the American Academy of Pediatrics. Web site addresses are as current as possible but may change at any time.

Brand names are furnished for identification purposes only. No endorsement of the manufacturers or products mentioned is implied.

The publishers have made every effort to trace the copyright holders for borrowed materials. If they have inadvertently overlooked any, they will be pleased to make the necessary arrangements at the first opportunity.

This publication has been developed by the American Academy of Pediatrics. The contributors are expert authorities in the field of pediatrics. No commercial involvement of any kind has been solicited or accepted in development of the content of this publication.

Every effort is made to keep *The Picky Eater Project: 6 Weeks to Happier, Healthier Family Mealtimes* consistent with the most recent advice and information available from the American Academy of Pediatrics.

Special discounts are available for bulk purchases of this publication. E-mail our Special Sales Department at aapsales@aap.org for more information.

Printed in the United States of America

9-367   1 2 3 4 5 6 7 8 9 10
CB0096

ISBN: 978-1-58110-981-8
eBook: 978-1-58110-982-5
Photography by Carl Tremblay
Cover and color insert designed by R. Scott Rattray
Library of Congress Control Number: 2015960361

What People Are Saying

The Picky Eater Project is a BRILLIANT solution to one of parenting's toughest dilemmas! Finally, an approachable, practical guide to the question "What's for dinner?" that instantly helps families, with children of all ages, conquer food phobias, get cooking, eat healthier, and, most of all, enjoy mealtime together!

Gail Simmons
Food expert, TV host, and author of *Talking With My Mouth Full*

—⁊⁊⁊—

Picky eating can cause family stress and can set up children for obesity and other health problems. Natalie Muth and Sally Sampson have ridden to the rescue with *The Picky Eater Project*. This practical book gives parents concrete steps to make mealtimes enjoyable and nutritious.

Christopher F. Bolling, MD, FAAP
Practicing pediatrician and Executive Committee Chair of the American Academy of Pediatrics Section on Obesity

—⁊⁊⁊—

This book sets the whole family up for fun cooking and eating at home with a plan that introduces the pleasure and the joy of tasting new foods. *The Picky Eater Project's* recipes are delicious, simple to prepare, and teach kids a new level of comfort in the kitchen that will be the basis for a lifetime of healthy eating.

Ana Sortun
Co-owner of Oleana, Sofra, and Sarma and author of *Spice*

—⁊⁊⁊—

—⌇⌇⌇—

This book is a recipe to defeat picky eaters. As Natalie and Sally suggest,
start early and steer kids toward variety, not toward picky eating.
I use these tips with my own kids and patients—
and they work.

Stephen Pont, MD, MPH, RDN, FAAP
Medical Director, Texas Center for the
Prevention and Treatment of Childhood Obesity

—⌇⌇⌇—

Muth and Sampson present a road map for parents to nurture food-literate
children—and also have some fun along the way.

Wendy Slusser, MD, MS, FAAP
Associate Vice Provost, UCLA Healthy Campus Initiative, where food literacy is
weaved into the fabric of the educational experience

—⌇⌇⌇—

For my husband, Bob, and children,
Thomas and Mariella.

Thank you for all of the joy you bring to my life.

– N. D. M.

To my children, Lauren and Ben,
who eat just about everything. And to everyone
at ChopChop Kids, who make all of this possible.

– S. S.

Contents

Note: All recipes in this book either appeared in ChopChop or are adapted from recipes in *The Fun Cooking Magazine for Families.*

Preface

My interest in kids' nutrition habits and especially picky eating piqued about a decade ago when I had recently completed my nutrition degree and training and was in medical school. I knew enough about nutrition and health to understand the recommendations of *what* kids *should* eat. But at the time, without kids of my own, I didn't fully appreciate the *how* of actually getting kids to eat healthy foods—foods such as bitter vegetables, which our taste buds as humans aren't really equipped to like at first. Spending one very stressful and unenjoyable lunch with my sister and her 2 young daughters was the event that set off my pursuit of wanting to understand and implement strategies that would help kids *want* to be healthy eaters and free parents of mealtime battles and struggles trying to force them to eat their vegetables.

My nieces were about 6 and 8 years old at the time. One liked to eat only carbohydrate foods such as pasta and white breads. The other one was a true carnivore and wanted to eat only protein-loaded foods such as meat and fish. Neither was much of a fan of fruits and vegetables. The only way that my sister could get them to eat in a more balanced way was through coercion and bribes. "Marion, eat some vegetables or you are not getting dessert." "Annie, you cannot just eat meat! Put some fruit on your plate. You are not getting up until you eat it." "Please just try one bite. You will like it. Just try it. Come on."

Not too long after that experience, it was my turn. My son, Thomas, was born in 2008. I knew I had just a couple of years until those battles would likely start brewing in my house unless I did something differently. The first couple of years with him were fairly easy. Like most kids, once he was about 6 months old and ready to begin solid foods, he eagerly ate anything I put in his mouth. But when he got to be about 18 months, he decided he was opposed to anything green. He didn't care so much for vegetables in general. Then he didn't really want much fish. No way would he try something spicy. With my son, I didn't know all the tools and techniques at first, despite my research. Since then, we've spent a lot of time undoing his picky eating, experimenting with different strategies that might work. The advice included in

The Picky Eater Project is the culmination of what research plus real-life experience with my son and the children of patients, family, and friends, plus all of Sally's personal experiences and work with *ChopChop* magazine and the kids it reaches, shows to work. I'm very happy to report that Thomas is now a much more adventurous eater than I ever imagined he would be when we were in the midst of his pickiness a few years back.

I learned some lessons throughout this journey. With my daughter, Mariella, who is 2 years younger than Thomas, we did things a little differently. Her Picky Eater Project started the day I knew I was pregnant. Between my 2 pregnancies I learned a lot. More research was published that showed we can take a lot of steps very early on to prevent picky eating, such as eating really interesting, flavorful, spicy, and bitter foods during pregnancy to expose the baby to the tastes in the amniotic fluid and continuing to eat those foods often during breastfeeding to further expose the infant. I did exactly that. Now 5 years old, willing to eat absolutely anything, and eager to make healthy choices, Mariella never experienced a picky phase. It might be part luck, but I think some of it is from my concerted efforts before she was even born. That is why we include tips for pregnancy and infancy in this book—because there is a LOT you can do to help prevent it from happening in the first place. But we know most readers are in the midst of picky eating with older kids and working to undo it, like I have done with Thomas. Here is all of our best advice based on current research to undo picky eating and bring some sanity back to mealtimes.

— Natalie Digate Muth

When I was in elementary school, the joke in our house was I ate only on Sundays, when my parents got lunch from a local deli.

Years later, when I was 14, I both expanded and contracted my diet by becoming a vegetarian, eating foods I can describe only as a far cry from what we got in the deli. My mother, a great and adventurous cook with a full-time job, told me she wasn't going to cook special food for me and I could eat the dinner she prepared, minus the meat. She wasn't angry but rather matter of fact: if I wanted something else, she said, I should learn to cook, which I did. In fact, it's probably why I became a cookbook writer.

Twenty-three years ago, I became a mother and had the same very laid-back attitude. Dinner was, and is, dinner. My 2 children mostly ate what we ate; I didn't cook 2 separate meals, never made them try anything, and didn't argue over their choices. I never hid a vegetable, I didn't use food as a carrot or a stick, and I didn't freak out if they didn't eat. But when their friends came over, it was a whole other story. This one wouldn't eat green food, that one wouldn't eat soft food, and on and on. We mostly used positive peer pressure and overall their friends ate the foods their parents swore they wouldn't eat.

Today, I run ChopChop Kids (www.chopchopkids.org), the nonprofit publisher of *ChopChop: The Fun Cooking Magazine for Families.* Our mission is to inspire and teach children to cook and eat real food with their families. I noticed whenever I spoke publicly about the value of cooking with kids, the bulk of the questions I got was about picky eating. More than anything it became what I talked about and ultimately became fascinated with. My answer is always cook with them.

Our hope is that this book will get you to the point where you cook with your kids on a regular basis. Teaching them to cook is a powerful tool in just about every way: it creates connections between generations, cultures, and places; teaches math, science, geography, and self-sufficiency; and is creative and fun.

Honestly, I feel like I've been on the same path my entire life. I believe most every child will enjoy most every healthy food, especially if they participate in its preparation.

— Sally Sampson

Acknowledgments

No book on how to help kids adopt healthy and adventurous palates would be complete without the tremendous experiences and contributions of kids and their families who have practiced the tips, experiments, and recipes included in this book, most especially *ChopChop* magazine readers; Christine, Fran, and their twins, Andrew and Nathaniel; and the stars of this book, Marlo, Corey, and their children, Brooke and Hunter. We are grateful for the energy and enthusiasm as well as the time and commitment all have devoted to not only working toward happier, healthier mealtimes for their families but also being willing to share their experiences in order to help other families achieve the same goal. In addition, we are forever indebted to our own families for their enthusiasm, good humor, flexibility, and ready acceptance of their role as guinea pig in trying out new ideas, recipes, and practical applications of research findings. I (N. D. M.) am also grateful to my great friend and sister, Nikki, and her 2 kids, Marion and Anneliese, whose mealtime battles sparked my interest in how to raise healthy eaters.

Thank you to Kathryn Sparks at the American Academy of Pediatrics who believed in the idea and brought us together to collaborate on this book and to the whole American Academy of Pediatrics publishing team and the pediatrician reviewers who support this project and helped make this book better. We'd also like to thank Dr David Ludgwig, who wrote the first Picky Eater series with Sally; KJ Dell'Antonia at the *New York Times,* who provided us a platform to share early findings of the Picky Eater Project on the Motherlode Blog (now Well Family); and our agent, Carla Glasser, for making possible this book, which we hope will help many families on their journey to happier, healthier family mealtimes.

Introduction

"People's tastes are not formed by accident."

— Brian Wansink, PhD, Cornell Food and Brand Lab

As moms to two kids each, as well as a cookbook author and founder of *ChopChop: The Fun Cooking Magazine for Families* (Sally), and a practicing pediatrician and registered dietitian (Natalie), we have worked with hundreds of families who are committed to raising their children to be healthy eaters. Along the way, almost all of them (including ourselves!) have had to deal with the very common experience of *picky eating.*

In fact, developing some pickiness is a normal part of childhood development. It is called "food neophobia"—the fear of trying new foods. Two-year-olds are infamous for it. For some kids it can stick around for a while—well into childhood and adolescence, and sometimes even adulthood. But it doesn't have to. While we may have some innate preferences for certain foods (especially sweet and salty), as Brian Wansink of the Cornell Food and Brand Lab summarizes in his 20 years of research on the subject, "[p]eople's tastes are not formed by accident."

Whether you are an expecting parent hoping to stave off picky eating (or undo your own picky preferences before your baby is born) or are the parent of an infant, a toddler, a school-aged child, or a teen, *The Picky Eater Project* offers you a week-by-week plan to help undo picky eating. It is more like having your own personal coach than reading a how-to guide. Each week, we focus on a key theme and then offer some guidance to help you develop your own plan to improve your family's nutrition and get creative in the kitchen while simultaneously slowly ticking away at picky eating preferences. Along the way, you'll also pick up some easy cooking tips and recipes, boost your family's overall well-being and harmony, and have fun at the same time! The tips and tricks from each chapter come to life with the authentic experiences of one family who has successfully completed the Picky Eater Project.

Get ready to embark on a journey that is certain to change the way you approach nutrition, mealtimes, and your relationship with your kids. For best results, we strongly recommend digging in and following the plan as a 6-week series and considering engaging your support system to help you include family members, friends (perhaps they'll want to do their own Picky Eater Project, too!), and your child's pediatrician. In a short period, you will see some big changes that will stay with you and your family over time. If later you come to a bump in the road, or if after 6 weeks you still aren't where you want to be, simply go through the process again (paying special attention to Chapter 8) and further reinforce your changes. Each week has a theme that builds upon the previous weeks. Here's a quick overview.

Chapter 1—Week 1: Picky-Free Parenting

First and foremost, picky eating is not your fault! Picky preferences are normal and expected and, as you may know firsthand, for some kids inherently very pronounced. While you cannot control what your child will and will not voluntary put into his or her mouth (and we definitely advise against force feeding your kids their vegetables and other healthy foods they refuse to eat!), you can take steps that will help your kids *want* to be more adventurous eaters. In the first week, we show you how with the **10 rules of "picky-free parenting."**

Chapter 2—Week 2: A Kitchen Revolution

Would your kids be totally content if they ate nothing other than pasta, white bread, macaroni and cheese, chicken nuggets, and other white, bland, and processed foods? Are your mealtimes stressful events where you try to convince your child to eat something with a little more color or variety? Or, maybe you've all but given up, preferring to let your kids eat what they want rather than fight about it or worry they will go to bed hungry. If so, you are not alone. In week 2, we show you ways to help your kids start to "train their taste buds" to start to like more flavorful, robust, and adventurous foods. And the best thing is, you don't have to say a word about it! No need to coerce, beg, or bribe them to try something new. Instead, we will show you how to change the way you purchase, arrange, and prepare foods so your kids try new foods without even realizing it. By putting your picky-free parenting into action, you will progress toward your vision of where you'd like your family to be with their eating habits by making a couple of key observations and setting and monitoring the progress of a few early goals.

Chapter 3—Week 3: The Little Cook

After more than 6 years of publishing *ChopChop* magazine and coaching hundreds of parents and children learning how to cook together, Sally knows firsthand the magic of involving kids in the kitchen, not only for helping them to become more adventurous eaters but also to gain critical life skills, bond with a parent, and just have fun! This week we practice inviting kids in the kitchen—ideally, early and often—and watch how the experience of cooking together helps a child train the taste buds to try new foods.

Chapter 4—Week 4: A Shopping Adventure

Life gets hectic, especially with kids, and especially those who are rigid in their eating preferences. While grocery shopping isn't usually what most people think of as a good time, this week we will work on developing grocery shopping as more of an adventure than a chore. We will also work to create easy-to-implement meal plans and grocery lists to help support the positive changes that have been occurring at home.

Chapter 5—Week 5: Family Mini-feast

The value of family meals includes, but extends far beyond, its role in helping children to acquire a taste for a wider variety of interesting foods. This week we strategize how to set up family meals to fit with your lifestyle while also reaping all of the benefits of eating together, including further progress in the pursuit of undoing picky eating. Meal and recipe ideas will give you the tools and guidance you need to put the plan into action.

Chapter 6—Week 6: It Takes a Village

By week 6 it will become abundantly clear that it would be difficult to make these changes alone. From a spouse or partner to the grandparents, siblings, and friends—everyone has a role to play. It takes a village to undo picky eating. This week we will work on the social support teams to help everyone own the change.

Chapter 7—Post–Picky Eater Project: Making It Stick-y

While your Picky Eater Project may officially be complete, we recommend going through our post–Picky Eater Project chapter to help make the changes stick. After all, we can do pretty much anything for a short period of time. But keeping it going for the long haul is imminently more challenging. In this chapter, we plan for challenges and barriers and put the contingency plans into action. Relapses happen. But how we respond to them determines how much of a lasting effect they will have. Just like any other behavioral change, we need a plan for making it stick.

Chapter 8—Troubleshooting

Despite all of your best efforts, you will run into challenges with keeping your Picky Eater Project going. And, in some cases, coexisting physical and mental health conditions can make it that much more challenging. What about food allergies? Sensory integration troubles? Medical diagnoses such as autistic spectrum disorder or feeding troubles? This chapter serves as a useful reference to identify and troubleshoot these and other challenges. In fact, if you are concerned that your child may have an underlying physical or mental health concern underlying his picky eating, we suggest you start the Picky Eater Project by reviewing this chapter first.

What You Can Expect

This book is very much intended to be an interactive guide rather than a book you sit down with, read in one sitting, and then put back on the shelf. You certainly will get the most out of the experience—and see the greatest payoff—if you practice the tools and techniques with your own kids and then reflect on the journey. To help you do this, we recommend a similar process for tackling each week.

1. Choose a goal or two for the week. See how this stacks up with your overall vision for what you hope to accomplish over the 6 weeks.
2. Pick two to three specific actions to take that week to meet the goal.
3. Come up with a plan to make those actions happen.
4. Follow through on the plan.
5. Make changes to the plan to make it work better.
6. Check in on your goals.

To help bring your Picky Eater Project to life, at the end of each week we will prompt you to consider the 6 steps outlined above in addition to suggesting activities and exercises for each week. You will also come across several features such as What's Your Story? and Try It Out games and experiments with prompts and tips to try the tactics at home and reflect on your experiences.

By the end, you will see how your family life has evolved over the 6 weeks of this Picky Eater Project. Mealtime food battles will be ancient history.

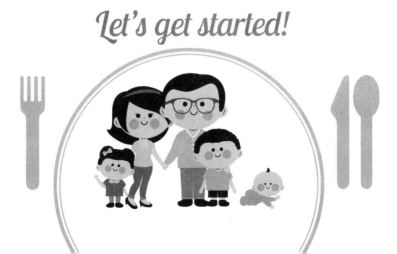

CHAPTER 1

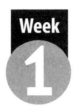

Picky-Free Parenting

No more
power struggle.
No more
mealtime battles.

Mission
Create more harmonious mealtimes.

Strategy
Practice 10 rules of "picky-free parenting."

Measurement
Number of pleasant mealtimes this week.

MEET THE FAMILY

Meet Marlo, Corey, Brooke, and Hunter.
Marlo and Corey reached out to us after another frustrating
night/week/month of wanting their kids to eat healthier but not feeling
like they had the tools they needed to make it happen and still maintain family
harmony. They graciously agreed to let us share their experiences to serve as an example
of how one family put the Picky Eater Project into action. As you follow along their
journey, you will witness firsthand their successes as well as their challenges.

the parents

Marlo is a nurse in a cardiac "cath lab." She loves to exercise and host get-togethers with family and friends. She is a self-described "people pleaser." She would really like to see her kids eat a greater variety of healthy foods, especially fish because she loves it and would like to make it for the family. Although she would like the kids to eat healthier, she'd rather they eat something (even if it's not very healthy or adventurous) than go to bed hungry because they are highly active and need the energy and calories to grow. Meal battles are not something she would prefer to fight about it. For this reason, she is happy to make 2 or more dinners to be sure all have something they will eat.

- **Marlo's all-time favorite foods:**
  sushi and pizza

- **Marlo's favorite vegetables:**
  artichokes and edamame

- **Marlo's least favorite foods:**
  broccoli and dark-meat chicken or lamb

- **Marlo's least favorite vegetables:**
  cilantro and broccoli

Corey is a federal agent and former Marine. He loves to surf and spend time with his kids. His goal is that the whole family eats one meal each night that everyone is willing to try (not the same acceptable meals day in and day out). It doesn't matter if the family meal is healthy (though he'd prefer that it be); he would just like everyone to agree on something.

- **Corey's all-time favorite food:**
  barbecue chicken thighs

- **Corey's favorite vegetable:**
  baked beans ("Does that count?")
  (Technically, beans are a vegetable and a protein, so we say **YES**, though baked beans typically have a considerable amount of added salt and sugar.)

- **Corey's least favorite food:**
  will eat anything

- **Corey's least favorite vegetable:**
  likes them all

MEET THE FAMILY

the kids

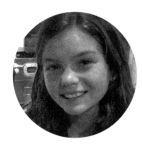 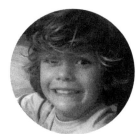

Brooke is 10 years old and in sixth grade. She loves swimming and spending time with her friends. Her goal is to flip a pancake without having it smear all over the pan and be trusted to use not just the microwave but also the oven, stove, and toaster. She is kind of excited to start the Picky Eater Project but also a little concerned. What exactly is it she's going to have to eat?

- **Brooke's all-time favorite foods:**
  turkey, stuffing, and cranberries

- **Brooke's favorite vegetables:**
  brocco-flower (never tried it but really wants to!) and celery

- **Brooke's least favorite food:**
  fish BUT she volunteers that she is open to eating salmon with "good sauce," which "tastes like a piece of candy"

- **Brooke's least favorite vegetable:**
  cauliflower ("It looks weird, but actually I might try to eat it.")

Hunter is 7 years old and in third grade. He loves baseball, swimming, math, and anything that involves being outside or requiring a lot of energy. His goal is to eat more artichokes. Despite being a picky eater, after hesitantly trying artichokes at a friend's house before the Picky Eater Project started, he learned he loves them and wants to eat them all the time.

- **Hunter's all-time favorite foods:**
  artichokes and pizza

- **Hunter's favorite vegetable:**
  artichokes

- **Hunter's least favorite food:**
  imitation crab

- **Hunter's least favorite vegetable:**
  None! He likes every kind of vegetable, though his parents say that is quite surprising since he won't eat most kinds of vegetables.

At the onset of their Picky Eater Project, we sat down with Marlo, Corey, and their kids, Brooke and Hunter, to better understand their family mealtime routines.

Family Schedule and Routine

Marlo has a very sporadic schedule, including many overnight and weekend calls.

Corey works as a federal agent with erratic but somewhat flexible hours. They co-parent, splitting most of the grocery shopping and meal prep. It turns out, as with many American families, it's quite a balancing act.

Hunter plays baseball and swims competitively. Brooke also swims competitively. Both kids are very high energy—especially Hunter—and love to be active.

There's not a lot of time to throw together gourmet meals, not that their kids would eat them anyway. Given Hunter's and Brooke's high level of physical activity and the understanding that kids need energy, vitamins, and minerals to grow, Marlo and Corey get anxious when their kids refuse to eat meals and are willing to make them something different just to be sure they eat enough, essentially often making 2 to 3 different meals at every mealtime.

GOAL: Their primary goal is to make one dinner for the whole family and additionally have the kids eat more vegetables (carrots are one of their favorites) and fish (they will not eat).

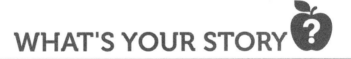

WHAT'S YOUR STORY

- How would you describe your family routines?
- How do your children's ages and activities and your career and priorities affect mealtimes at your house?
- Who is primarily responsible for selecting, purchasing, and preparing food at your house?

Meal Dilemma

Marlo and Corey usually start by offering one meal. But when their kids refuse it (which they do more often than not), they readily offer something else. Marlo and Corey would like their kids to be more adventurous in their eating choices, but do not feel it is worth fighting about or letting the kids "starve" by refusing to cook something else. Both agree that Brooke is the pickier of the two but also the most influential. If she tries something, Hunter will too. If she rejects it, there's little chance Hunter will go for it, unless he's trying to win "bonus points" with his parents.

Interestingly, when Brooke learned about the project, she jumped up, pulled an apron out of the kitchen drawer, and exclaimed, "Wait, does this mean I get to learn how to cook!" When Hunter learned of the project, he shared his disdain for Brussel sprouts but then, later, commented that if he helped make them and they looked like they would taste good, he would give them a try.

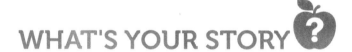

WHAT'S YOUR STORY

- What would you consider to be your greatest challenge during mealtimes?
- What parenting styles have helped or hurt as you've worked to help your kids eat a wider variety of foods?
- How did your kids respond when you told them you were going to be starting a Picky Eater Project at your house? If you haven't told them, why not?

Throughout a total of 6 weeks, Marlo, Corey, Brooke, and Hunter will serve as models of the Picky Eater Project in action. While the specific details of this family's experience will be different than what you experience, the process for undoing picky eating is the same, and we hope that looking on their experience will help your own Picky Eater Project come to life. Whether you have a toddler at her peak of pickiness or are struggling with persistently picky preferences in school-aged and teenaged kids, the Picky Eater Project will help you bring some sanity back to mealtimes.

As we advised to Marlo and Corey in their first week of the project, it is helpful to start with a vision of how you hope your kids' eating habits will turn out at the end of the day, once they're on their own (the ultimate test of this approach to raising healthy eaters), as well as what you hope to achieve by the end of the 6 weeks. Think of it kind of like your **family mission statement,** at least when it comes to food. This mealtime mission statement will serve as a compass to help prioritize your decisions and actions and align your everyday activities to the bigger picture.

For example, a mission statement could be as simple as
"We will be a family of adventurous eaters."

Or
"My children will grow up to be healthful eaters."

Or
"We will eat healthfully most days."

Or
"No more power struggle. No more mealtime battles."

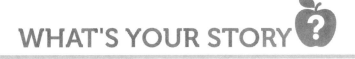

WHAT'S YOUR STORY

Write down a family mission statement. Post it someplace visible, where all family members can be reminded of it, throughout the 6 weeks of the Picky Eater Project.

Marlo and Corey's mission? To simply have a single meal at dinner.

What we suggested to Marlo and Corey, and suggest to all parents trying to avoid or reshape picky eating preferences, and realize their family mealtime mission, is to adopt a parenting style that we have coined "picky-free parenting." It is the middle ground between the hovering, micromanaging tendencies of a stereotypical helicopter parent (an authoritarian parenting approach) and the permissive, anything goes mentality of a stereotypical "free-range parent" (a permissive/hands-off or indulgent parenting approach). For example, when it comes to mealtimes, a helicopter parent might hover over a picky eater and demand that he eat everything on his plate or no dessert. A free-range parent might not mind if a child has loaded up on unhealthy foods—after all, that's better than starving. On the other hand, a picky-free parent will make sure a healthy, balanced meal is available most of the time and leave it to the child to choose what and how much of it to eat.

A picky-free style of parenting has also been referred to as "authoritative" or "responsive parenting." We prefer to use responsive parenting so as to avoid confusion between authoritarian and authoritative parenting. The idea is that parents set the stage for a child to feel empowered to make a choice and exercise some autonomy. The parents create structure and guidelines for their children but leave room for flexibility and negotiation. Children experience certain freedoms within well-described rules. In other words, the parent has been very strategic and thoughtful in setting the stage, so the child is highly likely to make a good choice.

What is your parenting style? Take the parent feeding quizzes (see Tables 1.1–1.4 on pages 9–11) to find out.

Are You a Picky-Free Parent? Child Feeding Questionnaire

Researchers developed the Child Feeding Questionnaire to better understand parents' strategies and ideas about child feeding. The questions on the next pages are excerpted from the full questionnaire and can help you determine if you tend to take a more free-range (permissive/indulgent), picky-free (authoritative/responsive), or helicopter (authoritarian) parenting approach to mealtimes.

Taking a picky-free approach to mealtimes, in which children are encouraged to eat healthy but also given some choices, is associated with improved nutrition and health outcomes. This is true even for picky eaters, whose parents may feel more invested in their nutritional choices and may have a tendency to practice a more authoritarian parenting style, which often turns out to be counterproductive. What is your parenting style? Take the parent feeding quizzes (Tables 1.1–1.4) to find out.

Table 1.1. Perceived Feeding Responsibility

Using the scale below, please circle one number for each question that best corresponds with your answer. Please answer with your child whose eating preferences you are most concerned about in mind.

	Never	Seldom	Half of Time	Most of Time	Always
1. When your child is at home, how often are you responsible for feeding your child?	1	2	3	4	5
2. How often are you responsible for deciding what your child's portion sizes are?	1	2	3	4	5
3. How often are you responsible for deciding if your child has eaten the right kinds of foods?	1	2	3	4	5

Table 1.2. Restriction

Using the scale below, please circle one number for each question that best corresponds with your answer. Please answer with your child whose eating preferences you are most concerned about in mind.

	Unconcerned	Slightly Unconcerned	Neutral	Slightly Concerned	Concerned
4. How concerned are you about your child eating too much when you are not around him/her?	1	2	3	4	5
5. How concerned are you about your child having to diet to maintain a desirable weight?	1	2	3	4	5
6. How concerned are you about your child becoming overweight?	1	2	3	4	5

Table 1.3. Pressure to Eat

Using the scale below, please circle one number for each question that best corresponds with your answer. Please answer with your child whose eating preferences you are most concerned about in mind.

	Disagree	Slightly Disagree	Neutral	Slightly Agree	Agree
7. I have to be sure my child does not eat too many sweets (eg, candy, ice cream, cake, pastries).	1	2	3	4	5
8. I have to be sure my child does not eat too many high-fat foods.	1	2	3	4	5
9. I have to be sure my child does not eat too many of his/her favorite foods.	1	2	3	4	5
10. I intentionally keep some foods out of my child's reach.	1	2	3	4	5
11. I offer sweets (eg, candy, ice cream, cake, pastries) to my child as a reward for good behavior.	1	2	3	4	5
12. I offer sweets (eg, candy, ice cream, cake, pastries) to my child as a reward for good behavior.	1	2	3	4	5
13. I offer my child his/her favorite foods in exchange for good behavior.	1	2	3	4	5
14. If I did not guide or regulate my child's eating, he/she would eat too many junk foods.	1	2	3	4	5
15. My child should always eat all the food on his/her plate.	1	2	3	4	5
16. I have to be especially careful to make sure my child eats enough.	1	2	3	4	5
17. If my child says, "I'm not hungry," I try to get him/her to eat anyway.	1	2	3	4	5
18. If I did not guide or regulate my child's eating, he/she would eat much less than he/she should.	1	2	3	4	5

Table 1.4. Monitoring

Using the scale below, please circle one number for each question that best corresponds with your answer. Please answer with your child whose eating preferences you are most concerned about in mind.

	Never	Rarely	Sometimes	Mostly	Always
19. How much do you keep track of the sweets (eg, candy, ice cream, cake, pastries) your child eats?	1	2	3	4	5
20. How much do you keep track of the snack foods (eg, potato chips like Doritos, cheese puffs) your child eats?	1	2	3	4	5
21. How much do you keep track of the high-fat foods your child eats?	1	2	3	4	5

Adapted with permission from Leann Birch. Original source: Birch LL, Fisher JO, Grimm-Thomas CN, Markey CN, Sawyer R, Johnson SL. Confirmatory factor analysis of the Child Feeding Questionnaire: a measure of parental attitudes, beliefs, and practices about child feeding and obesity proneness. *Appetite.* 2001;36(3):201–210.

Scoring

For each table, add your score.

Table 1.1. Perceived Feeding Responsibility

This measures the extent to which a parent feels a greater responsibility (versus a spouse or partner) for a child's nutritional intake, including portion sizes and types of foods eaten. *Total possible points:* 15.

Table 1.2. Restriction

This measures a parent's self-reported attempts to control a child's nutritional intake through restricting access to unwanted foods, including the types and amounts of those foods. *Total possible points:* 15.

Table 1.3. Pressure to Eat

These questions examine a parent's self-reported attempts to control a child's food intake, including the types and amounts of foods eaten. *Total possible points:* 60.

Table 1.4. Monitoring

This describes the extent to which a parent keeps track of a child's consumption of junk foods. *Total possible points:* 15.

In general, picky-free (responsive) parents tend to **score high** on perceived responsibility and monitoring and **low** on restriction and pressure to eat. On the other hand, helicopter (authoritarian) parents tend to **score high** on both restriction and pressure to eat, while free-range (permissive/indulgent) parents **score high** on restriction and **low** on monitoring.

So How Do You Put This Into Action?

Even if your natural tendency isn't along the lines of picky-free parenting, you can make small changes to your approach that will lead your family toward healthier, happier mealtimes. You've already created your family mission; now, we suggest creating your own family "rules" that the whole family will follow. Involve your kids in the process and post the rules on the refrigerator or in a common area where all

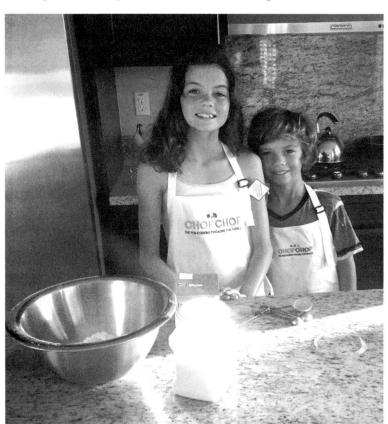

members of the family can be reminded of them. The more involved your children are in creating the family rules, the more likely they will be to follow them. If everyone agrees to follow the ground rules, it will be easy to come back and reinforce them.

10 Rules of Picky-Free Parenting

These are our suggested 10 rules of picky-free parenting. You may find you want to start with adopting some or all of them. Feel free to reword, restate, or elaborate on them to make them fit for your own family.

❶ As parents, we will be good role models. We will only ask the kids to eat foods that we are willing to eat ourselves.

❷ As parents, we will decide what foods are offered, when, and where. As kids, we will decide, of the food that is offered, what we will eat and how much.

❸ We will value the process of learning to be more adventurous eaters. We will be willing to try new foods, even if it is just a tiny bite.

❹ We do not have to clean our plates. We will listen to our bodies and let hunger be our guide.

❺ No food rewards will be offered. In other words, we kids do not have to "eat our vegetables" to get dessert on those days when dessert is available. We will not reward good behavior with sweets and "treats."

❻ Mealtimes equal family time. As often as we can, we will shop, cook, and eat together.

❼ We are one family, and we will eat one meal. We will not make separate meals. But we will be sure to include at least one thing each family member likes at most meals.

❽ We will learn together about food, nutrition, farming, and cooking.

❾ We will have fun, play, and experiment with new foods.

❿ We will be consistent in following these rules, but not rigid.

Table 1.5 offers some examples of picky-free parenting in practice based on a child's developmental stage.

Table 1.5. Picky-Free Parenting in Practice by Ages and Stages

Age/Stage	Picky-Free Parenting Tips	Recipe
Pregnancy	Make a habit of eating at least one unusual, new, or bitter food a few times per week. The flavors pass into the amniotic fluid and may help your baby be more willing to eat these foods down the road. Plus, the more you increase exposure to new foods, the more you will come to like them, and this will serve as modeling for your child down the road.	Cuban Black Bean Soup (For recipe, see page 21.)
Infancy	As a breastfeeding mom, eat a wide variety of unusual, new, or bitter foods a few (or more) times per week to help increase your baby's exposure to those foods through breast milk. **Adventurous solids** When introducing solids, when your infant is about 6 months old, introduce one new food at a time, with a special focus on bitter vegetables, a little bit of spice, and single-ingredient, adventurous foods. **Texture tasting** While you may start with purees, remember to advance texture over time to help a baby be willing to enjoy many different textures of foods. Once all the ingredients of a recipe have been introduced, it is fine to prepare them together. Infants have immature taste buds, which make them open to eating just about anything their first year or so of eating solid foods. As you advance textures, be sure the food is soft and small enough to prevent choking. Ultimately, by the time a child is 1 year old, she should be enjoying a wide variety of foods of varying smells, textures, and tastes—just like the rest of the family!	Baba Ghanoush (See page 23.)

Table 1.5 *(cont)*

Age/Stage	Picky-Free Parenting Tips	Recipe
Toddler	Age 2 is about when picky preferences (aka neophobia) kick in. Go with the flow while making it a habit to eat family meals together, and resist the temptations to force a child to eat or to cater to picky preferences or engage in mealtime battles. Instead, make sure at least one food your child likes is at each meal, and continue to provide a balanced meal, whether the child eats it or not.	Chicken Fingers (See page 25.)
Preschool	Engage your preschooler in the process of choosing and preparing foods. Kids are more likely to eat what they grow, choose, or prepare.	Tomato Salad With Basil and Feta Cheese (See page 26.)
School	Help your kids learn where their food comes from by growing a miniature garden. Plant easy-to-grow foods that the child might otherwise be resistant to try (eg, spinach, sweet peppers).	Mixed-up Eggs and Spinach (See page 27.)
Teen	Make a commitment to eat family meals together at least 2–3 times per week. This not only makes it more likely a teen will eat a balanced meal but also helps strengthen family relationships and decrease the likelihood of risk-taking behaviors. Require a teen to occasionally help choose and prepare meals to help him develop cooking skills. Require that the meal contain a protein, grain, fruit, and vegetable but otherwise avoid the urge to micromanage too much what the teen chooses.	Skillet Lasagna (See page 29.)

These rules will help support creating more harmonious, healthful mealtimes for your family. However, the mere existence of the rules will not be enough to change habits and behaviors. Box 1.1 shows how consistency and use of simple routines can help boost your kids' health. The rest of this book will help you translate these rules into normal family routines that will lead to healthier and happier mealtimes.

Box 1.1. How Simple, Consistent Routines Can Boost Kids' Health

Every parent wants to raise healthy, happy, stable kids. While there are certainly many ways to go about achieving this goal, implementing regular family routines has been shown, time and again, to help set the stage for raising successful kids. Mealtime, bedtime and screen time routines are associated with better nutrition, decreased risk of childhood obesity, improved child sleep (and parental sanity!), decreased risk-taking behaviors in teens, and fewer complications of chronic diseases such as asthma.

The Essential Components to Any Routine

The American Academy of Pediatrics published a report on actions families can take to help optimize child health. Establishing a successful routine was one of them, which the authors suggest is about more than enforcing a set dinner time or bedtime. The report suggests that for best results, a successful routine needs to include:

- A plan and scheduled time

- Elimination of distractions

- Direct communication of parental expectations

A Mealtime Example. A mealtime routine might include your family meal at 6:30 p.m. on weekdays, where your whole family sits together at the kitchen table. Television, phones and tablets are not allowed. At this time, each member of your family shares the best and worst parts of their days, and each one takes at least 20 minutes to eat together and reconnect with each other. No one is required to clean their plate, but all must remain at the table until they ask to be excused.

A Bedtime Example. A successful bedtime routine for your 5-year-old may start at 7 p.m. each night. It begins with a bath, followed by putting on pajamas and spending 15 minutes reading with a parent in a quiet room, with "screens" off and out of reach. You may then sing a short song and say "good night" to the child, remind the child that he or she is expected to go to sleep and not get out of bed until the morning comes, tuck the child into bed, give him or her a kiss on the forehead, and turn on the night-light before leaving the room.

Box 1.1 *(cont)*

A Screen Time Example. Many kids spend countless hours in front of screens playing video games, watching TV and staring at a computer or smartphone. In fact, many have established a habit of spending their afternoons with a screen rather than playing outside with their friends. Break this routine and create a new one by implementing a new screen-time rule. Plan ahead by choosing a set time of day in which screens are allowed, such as from 3:30-4:30 p.m. Make clear your expectation that they will not be eating or using multiple screens at one time during this hour. Share that outside of this one hour, you will not allow them to look at any kind of screen, and that you expect them to be doing something else— such as playing with their friends outside, doing homework or reading. Enforce this rule. (Author's note: The American Academy of Pediatrics recommends that children younger than 18 months to 2 years avoid screen time.)

Getting Started

Begin by simply taking inventory of your current routines. What would you like to see done differently? Choose just one routine, modify it and experiment to see how your family's daily experience changes. Once you've found a system that works, engage other influencers in your child's life. For example, does your child spend a significant amount of time with other caretakers? Aim to understand the routines your child has with them, and see if you can both adopt some of the same routines to help ease transitions.

Implementing these types of routines on a daily basis may seem overwhelming for busy families that struggle to simply get through the day, or that are rushing to shuttle kids from one practice to the next, with everyone on a different schedule. Yet, establishing routines helps to provide stability and a calm environment for kids, building their resilience and grit to withstand the chaos and pressures they may be feeling from the outside world.

Reproduced with permission from American Council on Exercise. Original source: Muth ND. Simple routines help boost kids' health. American Council on Exercise Family Health Web page. https://www.acefitness.org/acefit/healthy-living-article/59/3527/simple-routines-help-boost-kids-health. Published September 19, 2013. Accessed March 5, 2016.

YOUR PICKY EATER PROJECT—WEEK 1

Picky-Free Parenting

Project To-dos Checklist

☐ Draft a Family Mealtime Mission Statement.

☐ As a family, adopt your own family mealtime rules (see examples in 10 Rules of Picky-Free Parenting section on page 13).

☐ Complete the Child Feeding Questionnaire (see Tables 1.1–1.4 on pages 9–11).

☐ Setting out a specific vision helps achieve your mission. Start by answering the following questions: *What will success look like? In 6 weeks, 6 months, 6 years, 16 years?*

Resources

- Birch LL, Fisher JO, Grimm-Thomas CN, Markey CN, Sawyer R, Johnson SL. Confirmatory factor analysis of the Child Feeding Questionnaire: a measure of parental attitudes, beliefs, and practices about child feeding and obesity proneness. *Appetite.* 2001;36(3):201–210

- Fiese BH, Rhodes HG, Beardslee WR. Rapid changes in American family life: consequences for child health and pediatric practice. *Pediatrics.* 2013;132(3):552–559

- Hubbs-Tait L, Kennedy TS, Page MC, Topham GL, Harrist AW. Parental feeding practices predict authoritative, authoritarian, and permissive parenting styles. *J Am Dietetic Assoc.* 2008;108(7):1154–1161

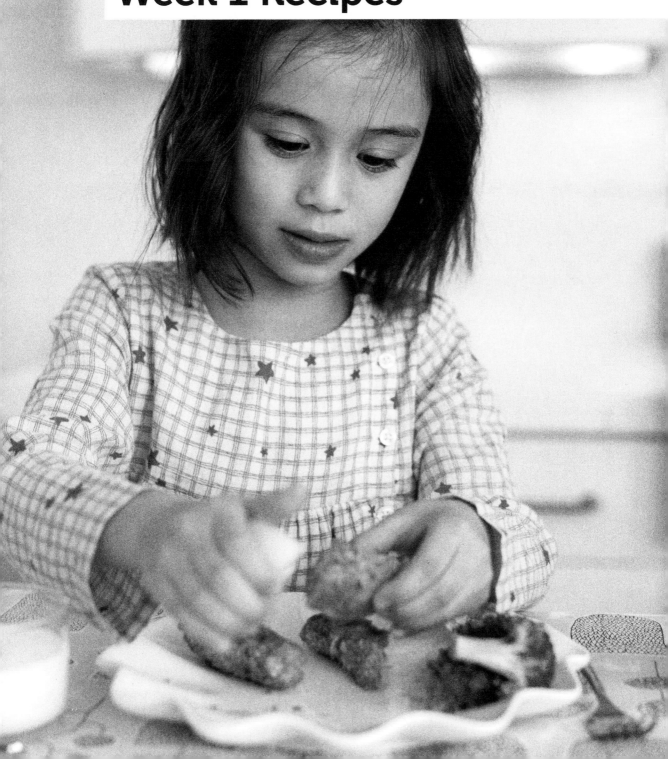

Week 1 Recipes

Cuban Black Bean Soup

Hands-on time: 30 minutes
Total time: 2 hours, 30 minutes
Makes: 10 cups

Rich in flavor and soft in texture, black beans, often called "black turtle beans," are perfect for soup. Black bean soup takes well to the classic Latin American flavors of cumin, chili, cilantro, and lime—add more or less of any of these, depending on what you like.

Kitchen Gear

Peeler

Can opener

Measuring spoons

Sharp knife

Cutting board

Colander or strainer

Measuring cup

Large heavy-bottomed pot

Wooden spoon or heatproof spatula

Pot holders

Ingredients

2 tablespoons olive oil

2 large onions, peeled and chopped

2 carrots, scrubbed or peeled, and chopped

2 celery stalks, chopped

4 garlic cloves, peeled, and minced or chopped

1 teaspoon ground cumin

1 teaspoon chili powder

1½ teaspoons dried oregano

1 teaspoon cayenne pepper (if you like it spicy)

3 (15-ounce) cans black beans, drained and rinsed

8 cups low-sodium chicken or vegetable broth

2 tablespoons fresh lime juice

½ cup chopped fresh cilantro leaves, for garnish

½ cup plain yogurt, for garnish

Instructions

1. Put the pot on the stove and turn the heat to medium. When it is hot, carefully add the oil.

2. Add the onions, carrots, celery, garlic, and spices and cook until tender, 10 to 15 minutes.

3. Add the beans and broth, raise the heat to high, and bring to a boil. Lower the heat to medium and cook partially covered for 2 hours, stirring frequently. (If at any point the soup seems too thick and is starting to look like mud, add 1 to 2 cups more broth.)

4. Just before serving, stir in the lime juice. Serve right away garnished with the cilantro and yogurt or cover and refrigerate up to 3 days.

Cuban Black Bean Soup *(cont)*

Kids in the Kitchen

- Teach your child how to measure ingredients and spices.

- Have your child rinse the beans using a colander or strainer.

- Your child can squeeze the lime for fresh lime juice.

- Ask your child to taste the soup: Does it need anything to boost the flavor? More spices? Another squeeze of lime juice? A grinding of black pepper? A pinch of salt? Add whatever you think it needs.

Personalize It

- Instead of lime juice, use lemon juice.

- Add 1 (16-ounce) can diced tomatoes.

- Swap in fresh basil leaves for the cilantro.

Baba Ghanoush

Hands-on time: 15 minutes
Total time: 1 hour, 15 minutes
Makes: 6 servings

Spread this herby, lemony dip on a sandwich; dollop it onto a salad; or scoop it up with raw vegetables, whole-grain crackers, or pita.

Kitchen Gear	**Ingredients**
Sharp knife	2 medium-sized eggplants
Cutting board	2 tablespoons olive oil
Measuring spoons	3 tablespoons fresh lemon juice
Rimmed baking sheet	2 garlic cloves, peeled and minced
Aluminum foil	2 tablespoons chopped fresh mint leaves or 1 teaspoon dried
2 forks	½ teaspoon salt
Pot holder	
Colander	
Food processor	
Serving bowl	

Instructions

1. Position the top oven rack about 10 inches above the heating element and set the oven to broil. Cover the baking sheet with aluminum foil.

2. Use a fork to prick each eggplant all over. Place them on the baking sheet and put the sheet in the oven. After 20 minutes, carefully take the baking sheet out of the oven and use 2 forks to turn each eggplant over. Place the baking sheet back in the oven, and broil the eggplants until they are completely collapsed and browned, about 25 additional minutes.

3. Place the eggplants in the colander and set aside to cool for 10 minutes. After they cool, use the 2 forks to turn each eggplant over. Allow them to drain, open side down, until they are cool enough to touch, about 15 minutes.

4. Pull the flesh from the skin. This is most easily accomplished with a fork and clean fingers, and will involve some combination of peeling the skin and scraping the flesh; be sure to get at all the nicely browned stuff right by the skin. Throw away the skin.

5. Put the eggplant flesh in the food processor fitted with the steel blade. Add the remaining ingredients and process until smooth, about 1 minute.

6. Scrape the dip into the bowl.

7. Serve right away or cover and refrigerate up to 2 days.

Baba Ghanoush *(cont)*

Kids in the Kitchen

- Let your child poke holes in the eggplant using a fork.

- Your child can squeeze the lemon for fresh lemon juice.

- Show your child how to separate the eggplant flesh from the skin.

- Let your child press the buttons on the food processor.

- Ask your child to taste the Baba Ghanoush: Does it need anything to boost the flavor? Does it need more lemon juice? More mint? A pinch of salt? If so, add it and, then, taste again.

Personalize It

- Instead of fresh mint, use fresh basil.

- Add 2 tablespoons tahini.

Chicken Fingers

Hands-on time: 10 minutes
Total time: 30 minutes
Makes: 4 servings

Oven-fried chicken is way better than pan-fried. It tastes better, is better for you, and doesn't smoke up the kitchen!

Kitchen Gear

Measuring spoons

Measuring cup

Sharp knife

Cutting board

Paper towel

Mixing spoon or whisk

Baking sheet

Large plate

Large bowl

Spatula or tongs

Ingredients

2 tablespoons olive or canola oil

1 cup fine bread crumbs or panko

½ cup whole-wheat flour

1 teaspoon kosher salt

½ teaspoon black pepper

¼ teaspoon cayenne pepper

2 large eggs, beaten

1 tablespoon Dijon mustard

1 teaspoon dried thyme

6 skinless chicken thighs, cut into thick strips

1 lemon, cut into quarters

Instructions

1. Turn the oven on and set it to 400 degrees Fahrenheit.

2. Pour the oil on the baking sheet and, using your clean hands or a paper towel, spread it around.

3. Place the bread crumbs, flour, salt, pepper, and cayenne on a large plate. Mix well.

4. Place the eggs, mustard, and thyme into the bowl and mix well. Add the chicken pieces and mix until they are well coated with the egg mixture.

5. Remove the chicken pieces one at a time from the egg mixture and let any extra egg mixture drip off.

6. Dip the chicken pieces one at a time in the bread crumb mixture, rolling them and pressing down to coat each side.

7. Shake off any extra coating; then put the chicken pieces on the baking sheet.

8. Transfer the baking sheet to the oven and bake for 15 minutes. Using a spatula or tongs, turn the chicken pieces over and bake until golden brown, 15 to 20 more minutes. Serve right away with a quarter of a lemon on each plate.

Tomato Salad With Basil and Feta Cheese

Hands-on time: 15 minutes
Total time: 10 minutes
Makes: 4 servings

Nothing says summer like a sun-warmed, fresh tomato you grew yourself. Buy a little pot of basil and leave it on your windowsill, or, better yet, if you have a garden, plant it.

Kitchen Gear
Sharp knife

Serrated knife

Cutting board

Measuring cup

Measuring spoons

Mixing bowl

Ingredients
4 large red tomatoes

½ cup crumbled feta cheese

2 tablespoons chopped fresh basil leaves

1 tablespoon olive oil

¼ teaspoon salt

Instructions
1. Use the sharp knife to remove the core from the tomatoes. Use the serrated knife to cut it into 1-inch cubes.
2. Combine the tomatoes, feta, and basil in a bowl.
3. Drizzle with the olive oil and sprinkle with the salt.
4. Serve right away or cover and refrigerate up to overnight.

Personalize It
- Instead of feta, use diced mozzarella, cheddar, or grated Parmesan cheese.
- Add ½ teaspoon curry powder.
- Swap in fresh peaches or nectarines, pitted and diced, for 2 of the tomatoes.
- Add 1 to 2 cups white beans or chickpeas.

Kids in the Kitchen
- Count the tomatoes.
- Let your child mix everything together.
- Ask your child to taste the salad: Does it need anything to boost the flavor? Does it need more basil? A pinch of salt? If so, add it and, then, taste again.

Mixed-up Eggs and Spinach

Hands-on time: 20 minutes
Total time: 20 minutes
Makes: 2 servings

Kitchen Gear

Measuring cup

Sharp knife

Cutting board

Measuring spoons

Medium-sized bowl

Fork or whisk

Skillet

Heatproof spatula

2 plates

Ingredients

4 large eggs

1 cup flat-leaf spinach, rinsed well and finely chopped

2 tablespoons chopped scallion greens and whites

½ teaspoon salt

1 tablespoon olive oil

Instructions

1. Crack the eggs into the bowl and mix well.

2. Add the spinach, scallions, and salt and mix again. (The mixture will look very spinachy and not very eggy.)

3. Place the skillet on the stove and turn the heat to medium. When the skillet is hot, carefully add the oil.

4. Add the egg mixture and let it cook for 1 to 2 minutes. Start carefully flipping portions of the eggs, so that you do not fully scramble the eggs but rather gently toss them.

5. When fully cooked (no more runny-looking egg), divide the eggs between the 2 plates. Serve right away.

Mixed-up Eggs and Spinach *(cont)*

Personalize It

Add other vegetables to your eggs, such as

- Chopped peppers

- Chopped onions

- Chopped broccoli

Kids in the Kitchen

- Have your child practice whisking the eggs with a whisk or fork.

- Let your child stir and flip the egg mixture while in the skillet.

- Ask your child to taste the eggs: Do they need anything to boost the flavor? Do they need a pinch of salt? If so, add it and, then, taste again.

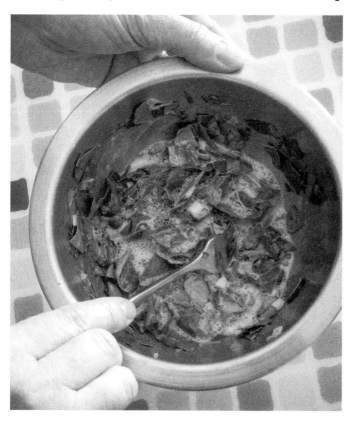

Skillet Lasagna

Hands-on time: 1 hour
Total time: 1 hour, 30 minutes
Makes: 6 servings

Everybody loves lasagna, and our fuss-free recipe makes it easy: the pasta and sauce layer beautifully without a lot of effort on your part. Just make sure to keep the heat low so the noodles cook through without the bottom burning. You can make the sauce ahead of time. Simply reheat it and proceed with the recipe.

Kitchen Gear

Measuring spoons

Sharp knife

Cutting board

Measuring cup

Can opener

Box grater

Large (10-inch) skillet with lid

Heatproof spatula

Ingredients

1 tablespoon olive oil or vegetable oil

1 large onion, chopped

1 garlic clove, peeled and minced

2 zucchini, ends trimmed, diced

1 teaspoon dried basil or oregano

1 (28-ounce) can diced tomatoes, including liquid

1½ cups water

2 cups fresh flat-leaf spinach leaves, coarsely chopped

8 no-boil lasagna noodles, broken in half

1 cup ricotta cheese

1 cup freshly grated Parmesan cheese

1 cup shredded mozzarella or Monterey Jack cheese

½ cup chopped fresh basil leaves

Skillet Lasagna *(cont)*

Instructions

1. To make the sauce, place the skillet on the stove and turn the heat to medium-low. When the skillet is hot, carefully add the oil. Add the onion and garlic and cook, stirring frequently, until tender, about 10 to 15 minutes.

2. Add the zucchini and basil or oregano and cook covered until the zucchini is just golden and tender, about 10 to 15 minutes.

3. Add the tomatoes and water and stir well. Turn the heat down to low and cook covered for 10 minutes. Remove the lid and cook an additional 10 minutes.

4. Turn the heat off. Add the spinach and stir until the spinach is wilted.

5. Carefully slip 4 noodle pieces into the skillet, using their edges to slide them under the bottom of the sauce, and using the spatula, push them down below the surface. Layer on another 4 noodle pieces and then another 4 and push them all below the surface. Add the last 4 noodle pieces and spoon a little bit of the tomato mixture on top.

6. Add the ricotta 1 tablespoon at a time, dotting the top with dollops. Sprinkle on the mozzarella or Monterey Jack, and then Parmesan cheese.

7. Reheat the skillet over low heat, cover, and continue cooking until the cheeses melt and the noodles are tender when you poke them with the tip of a knife, about 20 minutes. Sprinkle with the basil leaves. Set aside 10 minutes.

8. Serve right away or cover and refrigerate up to 2 days.

Kids in the Kitchen

- Show your child how to measure and chop ingredients, herbs, and spices.
- Have your child use a can opener to open the can of tomatoes—keep an eye out for sharp edges!
- Have your child break the lasagna noodles.
- Have your child add dollops of ricotta and sprinkle Parmesan, and mozzarella or Monterey Jack cheese.

Personalize It

- Eliminate the zucchini.
- Substitute 2 cups mushrooms for the zucchini.
- Substitute baby kale for the spinach.
- Instead of mozzarella cheese, use fontina.

CHAPTER 2

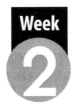

A Kitchen Revolution

"A choice architect has the
responsibility for organizing
the context in which people
make decisions."

—Richard H. Thaler,
*Nudge: Improving Decisions
About Health, Wealth,
and Happiness*

Mission
Create an environment that supports
more adventurous eating.

Strategy
Transform the kitchen—what is available,
where, when, and how.

Measurement
How many times kids try a new food of their choice
with no pressure.

Rows of ramen noodles, cheese crackers, chips, granola bars, canned soup, brownie mix, and a variety of other packaged foods lined the pantry shelves. Tucked away in a corner were pistachios, seaweed snacks, water, and a few other whole-grain snacks. The refrigerator included last night's leftovers, some vegetables, milk, juice, and some fruit hidden away in the lower drawers. The freezer was stocked with frozen chicken nuggets, ice cream bars, and a good variety of frozen vegetables and meats. As we went through the pantry and refrigerator, Marlo reflected: "I wish we could all eat better together. They don't like the food that I like. I don't like the food that they like. So we end up eating a bunch of different meals when we sit together at night."

Our advice was simple: think about the foods you want your family to eat, get rid of everything else, and stock your pantry and refrigerator with those foods. Easy to say, but how exactly do you do it? And what will be the repercussions when some of the kids' favorite foods are gone?

Our strategy for week 2 is to help kids be more interested in trying new foods by making it really, really easy to choose to eat them. We do that through a refrigerator, pantry, and countertop makeover. The idea is that the healthy foods become highly accessible and therefore easy to choose and the unhealthy foods become hard to find and easy to forget about.

Marlo took our advice to clean out the refrigerator, pantry, and countertop to heart, although it wasn't easy. She dumped the highly processed foods; bought healthier snack packs, such as unsalted nuts; and filled the refrigerator with vegetables and fruits, which she placed at the kids' eye levels. Not-so-healthy foods she or other family members couldn't part with she tucked away in a hard-to-find corner of the pantry, refrigerator, or freezer. She said nothing else about it, and while the kids didn't really seem to notice, they also proceeded to eat the food that was most available to them, including more fruits and vegetables. Marlo made her kitchen revolution pay off in a big way for her school-aged kids. You can, too. Check out our tips by age and stage in Table 2.1 for more advice on how to make this work for your family.

WHAT'S YOUR STORY ❓

- Take a quick look in your own pantry and refrigerator. What foods are front and center? Are they generally healthy or not so much?

- Ask yourself: If your kids all of a sudden decided they wanted to eat 5 servings of fruits and vegetables today, would you have enough of these foods in your house for them to do that?

- What do you think will happen if you completely reorganize your refrigerator and pantry? How will your kids respond?

Table 2.1. How to Make Your Kitchen Revolution Work by Age and Stage

Age/Stage	Kitchen Revolution Tips	Recipe
Pregnancy	Buy a new food this week that you've never tried before. Whether it is a strange new vegetable (ever tried jicama or turnips?) or a new type of pepper or spice, even though as a rule you may not like spicy food. Store it front and center in your refrigerator, in the pantry, or on the countertop, and seek out a recipe to use it in sometime this week. Just like the bitterness of coffee and tea is learned, so is liking previously rejected foods. Remember, it can take up to 20 times of trying it before you have retrained your taste buds.	Spicy Turkey Chili (For recipe, see page 54.)
Infancy	(Most) babies love to try new foods! Make a commitment to buy a new food that your baby has never tried—or that older kids refuse to eat (eg, a green vegetable)—and incorporate it into a homemade baby puree. Ask your older kids if they would like to give this experiment a try too!	Sweet Potato Spinach Baby Puree (See page 56.)
Toddler	Now that you have an abundance of healthy foods stocked in your kitchen, it's a great time to encourage your toddler to explore the different tastes. Toddlers are especially open to trying foods put together in fun and creative ways and any food that involves dip. Try veggie sticks in a plastic baggie decorated with stickers or a fun arrangement of colorful foods.	Parmesan Yogurt Dip With Carrots or Layered Yogurt Parfait (See pages 53 and 59.)

Table 2.1 *(cont)*

Age/Stage	Kitchen Revolution Tips	Recipe
Preschool	Preschoolers love when they get to help choose and make foods. Let them pick what vegetable to have with dinner, take them along when you go grocery shopping, and make it a family project to plant a few seeds (preschoolers generally love to eat what they grow). Make sure you (and other adults in the house) have a healthy and positive attitude toward vegetables and fruits. Also, strategize with the parents of your child's closest friends—does your son not eat a vegetable that his best friend loves? Have his best friend's mom or dad offer it up at their next playdate. With time, you might find that food on your child's list of favorites.	Roasted Vegetables (See page 57.)
School	Undoing picky eating can be hard for school-aged children because they already have somewhat established eating preferences. If you give the option between a salty processed snack and a fruit or vegetable, most are going to choose the salty snack every time. So don't give them that choice. Instead, offer a choice between 2 healthy options, or simply place a healthy snack on the table and let them decide whether or not to try it, but make sure that the unhealthy snack is not available as an alternative option. At mealtimes, make small changes to already preferred meals to make them a little bit healthier. For example, the chicken/turkey/pork/lamb burgers recipe in this chapter offers a healthy alternative to a standard hamburger.	Every Kind of Burger (Well, Almost) (See page 60.)
Teen	Your kitchen redesign will likely have the greatest effect for your teens. Teens are growing rapidly and need energy and calories to fuel that growth. That means they'll eat pretty much whatever is available. After you dump the junk food, when they are at home your teens will have no option but to eat the healthy food you've stocked up. Or better yet, get the teens in the kitchen to try it out for themselves.	Energy Bars (See page 62.)

Kitchen Revolution Guidelines

First: The Fridge

Nudge your family toward healthier choices by storing the healthy foods front and center and the less healthy foods, or the preferred foods you wish your child would eat less of, in harder-to-see places. Here's how.

❶ **Clean it out.** It is best to get on a schedule and do this weekly to minimize food spoilage and keep your refrigerator clutter-free. Remove everything from the refrigerator, give the shelves a good cleaning, and trash any expired foods or items that no one is likely to ever eat.

❷ **Take inventory.** Make a list of food you need to purchase to be able to prepare your planned meals for the week. Planned meals are generally healthier with less food wasted.

❸ **Now, *strategically* restock.**
- **Not-so-close.** Put the not-so-healthy items in the back of the refrigerator. This way, you and your family will have to work a little bit to find and eat them. That one extra step will go a long way in those foods being eaten less frequently.

- **Front and center.** Put the fruits and vegetables on the main shelves in the refrigerator. We have all had healthy produce go bad because we forgot about it in a fruit and vegetable drawer. If you put them in a location that can't be missed, you and the family will be more likely to eat them.

- **Prepare.** If you prep the healthy stuff, it is more likely to be eaten. Thoroughly wash fruits and vegetables and cut them into snack-sized pieces. Put them in clear containers so they won't be missed.

- **No waste.** Place leftovers and food that needs to be eaten soon in an easy-to-find location. Plan to use leftovers for lunches and snacks. For example, use leftover chicken in salads and sandwiches instead of prepackaged and not-so-healthy (due to high sodium and nitrites) deli meat.

- **Milk, water, iced tea (oh, my!).** Minimize space for unhealthy drinks. Try to include only fat-free milk, water, iced tea (for the adults; caffeinated drinks are generally not recommended for kids), or other beverages that are low in calories in the refrigerator. If the less healthy beverages like sodas and juice boxes are a normal part of your family's day and you aren't ready to avoid them, try to decrease consumption by keeping only single-serving amounts in the refrigerator for now. In the long run, if you can ditch the sugary drinks, the whole family will benefit tremendously.

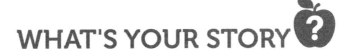

WHAT'S YOUR STORY

- Which were the easiest items to throw out? Which were the hardest?
- Did you make a list of planned meals for the week and take inventory of the items you needed to buy to make those meals? If so, how confident are you that you will follow your list? What would you need to increase your confidence?
- How does your post-makeover fridge look different than your pre-makeover fridge?

Next: The Pantry

The food available in your pantry can make or break your Picky Eater Project. You will eat much healthier by default when you stock your pantry in a way that makes eating a variety of healthy foods easy. Here's how.

❶ **Empty it out.** Start your pantry makeover by completely emptying it out. This will not only help you identify the types of food that you have accumulated but also set the stage for getting rid of unhealthy foods and clutter from the pantry. This is also a great time to remodel or reorganize your pantry to make it more attractive and user-friendly.

❷ **Pitch and toss.** Throw away all outdated or expired food and packaged food that contains any variation of sugar as the first or second ingredient or more than 13 grams of added sugar per serving (Table 2.2). Do the same with high-sodium products— does a single serving of chips provide almost half of your child's recommended sodium level? Toss it. It is OK to hold on to items you can't toss because you need to use them occasionally (eg, brown or granulated sugar) or foods you just aren't ready to part with, but when you restock the pantry, store these items in harder-to-see-and-reach places.

Table 2.2. All the Ways to Say Sugar

Sugar comes in many forms on the ingredient list. These words are all variations of sugar.

Agave nectar	Evaporated cane juice	Malt syrup
Brown sugar	Fructose	Maple syrup
Cane crystals	Fruit juice concentrates	Molasses
Cane sugar	Glucose	Raw sugar
Corn sweetener	High-fructose corn syrup	Sucrose
Corn syrup	Honey	Syrup
Crystalline fructose	Invert sugar	
Dextrose	Maltose	

Table 2.3. Characteristics of Healthy Snack Options

Nutrient Qualities	Sample Snacks
Is either Fruit Vegetable Whole grain Fat-free or low-fat milk product Fish Extra-lean meat or poultry Eggs Nuts or seeds Beans	• Any fresh, frozen, dried, canned, or baked vegetable or fruit • Whole-grain crackers • Almonds, walnuts, cashews, or peanuts • Plain yogurt • Canned tuna or salmon • Low-fat cheese slice or cheese stick • Hard-boiled egg
The healthiest snacks contain Less than 15% of calories from saturated fat and no trans fat No more than 13 grams of added sugars per serving Less than 210 milligrams of sodium per serving	

Derived from Federal Trade Commission, Centers for Disease Control and Prevention, US Food and Drug Administration, US Department of Agriculture. *Interagency Working Group on Foods Marketed to Children: Preliminary Proposed Nutrition Principles to Guide Industry Self-Regulatory Efforts; Request for Comments.* Center for Science in the Public Interest Web site. https://cspinet.org/new/pdf/IWG_food_marketing_proposed_guidelines_4.11.pdf. Accessed April 1, 2016.

❸ **Restock.** Now, restock with the good stuff. Check out Table 2.3 for expert recommendations to help identify snacks and meals for the kids that are generally healthy. Use our Picky Eater Project Pantry Guide (Box 2.1) for specific suggestions on foods to include.

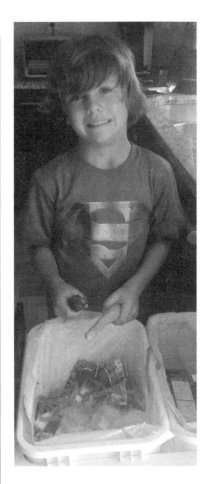

Box 2.1. The Picky Eater Project Pantry Guide

Stock your pantry with these food items to optimize your family's health and make sure you have all the essentials on hand when you need them.

Canned vegetables, beans, and fruits. These canned products can be just as healthy as their fresh counterparts if you purchase low-sodium variations for the vegetables and rinse with water before cooking. For fruits, choose canned fruit that lists it in its own juice.

Nuts and seeds. Have reduced-salt nuts and seeds on hand to add to meals and salads, as well as for snacking. Walnuts, almonds, pine nuts, pistachios, and cashews are excellent additions to any pantry. Try to avoid beer nuts, high-salt mixed nuts packages, and macadamia nuts.

Pastas and grains. Make sure to include whole-grain and high-fiber pastas and grains in your pantry. Brown rice, couscous, bulgur, oatmeal, barley, buckwheat, and quinoa are just a few examples of health-boosting grains. Transition from white pasta and flour to the whole-grain versions to boost health.

Herbs, spices, and oils. A mix of spices, dried herbs, and oils will help liven your cooking. Spices and dried herbs generally have a shelf life of 1–2 years. Check the flavor and color of spices to see if they are still up to par to meet your cooking needs (old spices won't be very flavorful, but they also won't make you sick). Make sure you have plenty of heart-healthy olive oil and canola oil on hand.

Finally: The Countertop

You can decrease kitchen clutter and increase the number of fruits, vegetables, and other healthy foods your family eats by reengineering how you organize, decorate, and use kitchen countertops and the kitchen table.

❶ Clean the clutter. Decrease your kitchen clutter by cleaning off the countertops and kitchen table and relocating the "stuff" to a file box or by creating an organization system. Likewise, if a variety of small kitchen appliances like a blender, toaster, or coffeemaker or other gadgets have filled your countertops, try to clear some shelf space for them. Do you keep a cookie container, candy bowl, or other highly visible and not-so-healthy snack on your countertops or tables? We suggest you move it out of sight.

❷ Fruit for thought. Reorganize the counter space in a way that promotes a healthy kitchen. Start with a bowl of fresh fruit. Place it in a highly trafficked area and your family's fruit consumption will increase immediately. Not so sure? See for yourself with our kitchen traffic experiment (Try It Out: The Kitchen Traffic Experiment).

TRY IT OUT

The Kitchen Traffic Experiment

The Hypothesis

When children frequently see and pass by healthy foods placed strategically in high-traffic areas such as a kitchen island, a table, or an eye-level shelf in the pantry, they will eat more of that healthy food.

The Experiment

Part A. Place a predetermined number of an easy-to-eat fruit in its normal location in your home. Each night before going to bed, count how much of the fruit has been eaten. Do this for 3 days.

Part B. Then for the next 3 days, place the same amount of the same fruit in a high-traffic area. Again, each night before going to bed, count how much of the fruit has been eaten.

Compare the results from parts **A** and **B.** What did you find?

❸ Growing a healthy interest. Get the kids on board to help you plant (or buy) an indoor herb garden. It may be just a few staples, like basil and oregano, or you could be more elaborate (see the Lowdown on Herbs and Spices section below for a quick overview of commonly used [and not so commonly used] herbs and spices). People (especially kids) love to eat what they grow. This small and easy-to-care-for garden will increase healthy food consumption and help liven home-cooked meals.

The Lowdown on Herbs and Spices

When it comes to feeding the family healthy foods that they'll actually eat, you can't go wrong with herbs and spices. For starters, herbs are easy to grow in temperate climates (spices are a little more difficult since they tend to originate in specific climates). You can set up a windowsill or backyard garden and grow a wide variety of greens. Kids tend to eat what they grow, which increases the odds they'll be willing to give the food a chance. Second, herbs bring a blast of flavor to foods, thus increasing the taste without having to load on the calories and salt. Who doesn't like to eat what tastes good? Finally, herbs and spices are loaded with nutrients, giving your health a boost, too.

You can mix and match herbs and spices to transform healthy, but bland, meals (like grilled chicken breast and steamed vegetables) into a cultural masterpiece. For instance, use the following herb and spice combinations to give a basic meal a distinct and delicious flare:

- **Indian:** garlic + onion + curry powder + cinnamon

- **Asian:** garlic + scallions + sesame + ginger + soy sauce

- **Italian:** garlic + basil + parsley + oregano

- **Middle Eastern:** garlic + onion + mint + cumin + saffron + lemon

- **Mexican:** cumin + onion + oregano + cilantro

So, how well do you know your herbs and spices? In the alphabetized list below, see how many you recognize and then learn where each comes from and what they're used for.

- **Allspice,** berry of the evergreen "pimento tree"; commonly used in Jamaican cooking. Tastes like a mix of cinnamon, nutmeg and cloves, thus the name "allspice."

  Uses: chicken, beef, fish (key ingredient in "jerk" dishes), fruit desserts, cakes, cookies, apple cider.

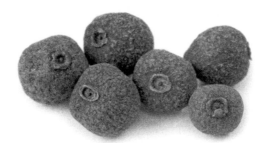

- **Basil,** aromatic leaf of the bay laurel. Pungently aromatic, sweet, spicy flavor.

  Uses: essential ingredient in Italian and Thai dishes; main ingredient in pesto.

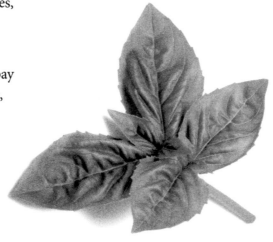

- **Bay leaf,** leaf of evergreen laurel. Aromatic, bitter, spicy, pungent flavor.

  Uses: soups, stews, braises and pâtés; used often in Mediterranean cuisine.

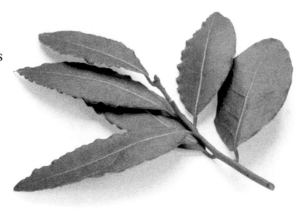

- **Caraway seed,** fruit of biennial herb of parsley family. Warm, biting, acrid but pleasant, slightly minty.

  Uses: rye breads, baked goods; often used in European cuisine.

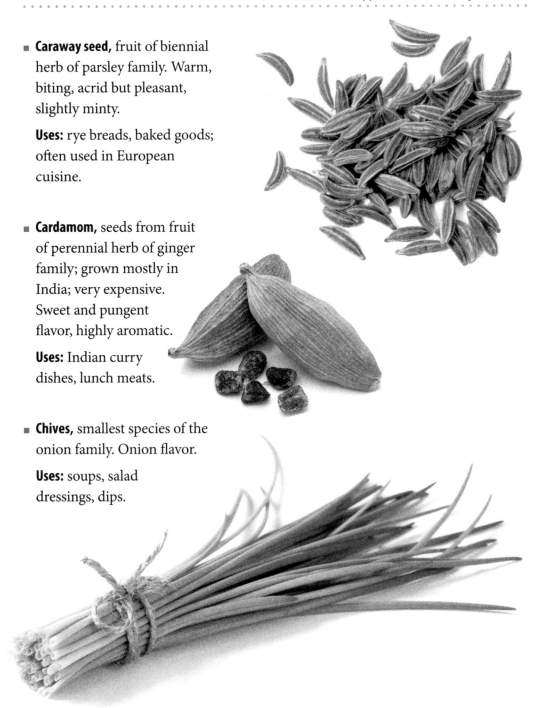

- **Cardamom,** seeds from fruit of perennial herb of ginger family; grown mostly in India; very expensive. Sweet and pungent flavor, highly aromatic.

  Uses: Indian curry dishes, lunch meats.

- **Chives,** smallest species of the onion family. Onion flavor.

  Uses: soups, salad dressings, dips.

- **Cilantro (coriander),** annual flowering herb, can be cultivated for leaves, seeds, flower, and roots. May have "soapy" versus "herby" taste, based on genetics of taster.

  Uses: often used in Latin American, Indian and Chinese dishes; in salsa and guacamole, stir fry, grilled chicken or fish; best when used fresh.

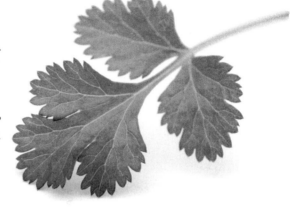

- **Cloves,** dried flower buds from evergreen of myrtle family. Warm, spicy, astringent, fruity, slightly bitter flavor.

  Uses: whole cloves on ham or pork roast; ground cloves to season pear or apple desserts, beets, beans, tomatoes, squash and sweet potatoes.

- **Cumin seed,** seeds of flowering plant of parsley family. Earthy and warming flavor.

  Uses: curry powder, chilies, used throughout world (second most common seasoning after black ground pepper).

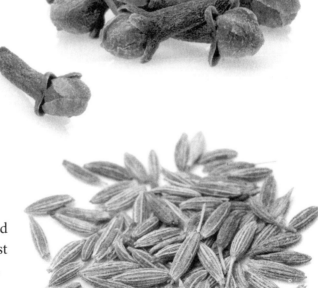

- **Ginger,** underground stem of perennial tropical plant. Biting flavor, fragrant.

  Uses: Asian dishes, marinade for chicken and fish, gingerbread, cookies, processed meats.

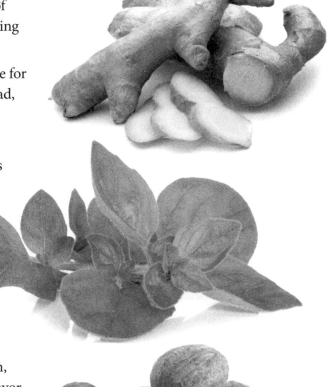

- **Marjoram,** leaves and flowers of perennial of mint family. Sweet pine and citrus flavor.

  Uses: meats, fish, poultry, vegetables, soups.

- **Nutmeg,** seed of fruit of evergreen tree. Sweet, warm, pungent, aromatic, bitter flavor.

  Uses: eggnog, French toast, cooked fruits, sweet potatoes, spinach.

- **Oregano,** leaves of perennial of the mint family. Related to marjoram, but very different flavor. Strong, pungent, aromatic, bitter flavor.

  Uses: Italian dishes, chili, beef stew, pork and vegetables.

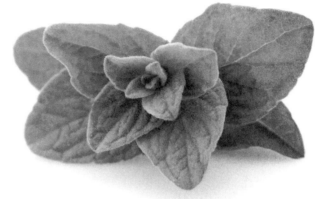

- **Parsley,** leaves of a biennial herbaceous plant; curly and flat leaf varieties. Grassy, bitter flavor.

  Uses: widely used throughout world, including in meat, soup, vegetables; often used as garnish.

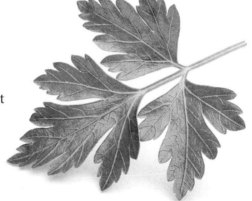

- **Rosemary,** woody perennial herb of evergreen shrub of mint family. Sweet, spicy, peppery flavor.

  Uses: flavoring in stuffing and roast lamb, pork, chicken and turkey.

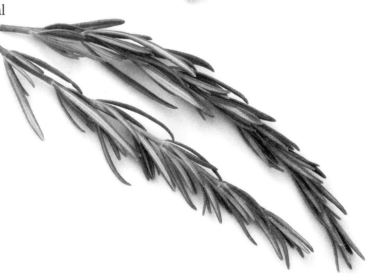

■ **Saffron,** spice derived from flower of iris family; very expensive. Earthy, sweet flavor.

Uses: baked goods, rice dishes.

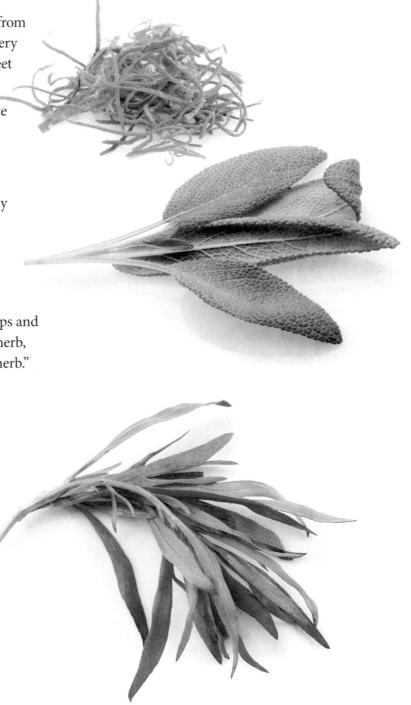

■ **Sage,** medicinal plant of mint family. Slightly peppery flavor.

Uses: often used to flavor fatty meals.

■ **Tarragon,** flowering tops and leaves of a perennial herb, often called "dragon herb." Minty "anise-like" (resembles licorice) flavor.

Uses: chicken, fish, egg dishes; one of four fines herbes of French cooking.

- **Thyme,** leaves and flowering tops of a shrub-like perennial of the mint family. Biting, sharp, spicy, herbaceous flavor; blends well with other herbs.

  Uses: meats, soups and stews.

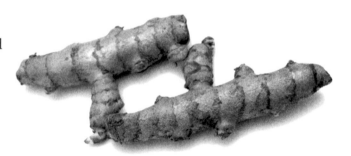

- **Turmeric,** stem of plant of tropical perennial herb. Mild, peppery, mustardy, pungent taste.

  Uses: curry powders, mustards, condiments.

Reproduced with permission from Healthy Learning. Original source: Muth ND. *Eat Your Vegetables! and Other Mistakes Parents Make: Redefining How to Raise Healthy Eaters.* Monterrey, CA: Healthy Learning; 2012.

YOUR PICKY EATER PROJECT—WEEK 2

A Kitchen Revolution

Project To-dos Checklist

☐ Remove your selective eater's highly preferred, not-so-healthy foods from the house this week. Give your child the option to choose anything else available in the home that he'd like to eat, and let him help you prepare it for the whole family.

How did it go?

☐ Embark on the kitchen makeover and restock your refrigerator and pantry with just the foods you need for the week, based on your meal plan and shopping list.

☐ Together with your selective eater, plant a mini herb garden in your backyard or windowsill.

☐ Try the kitchen traffic experiment (see Try It Out: The Kitchen Traffic Experiment on page 40).

What happened?

How might you modify the experiment for an even greater effect, or to broaden your child's food interests further?

Project Check-in: Remembering the Bigger Picture Goals

❶ What was your major goal for this 6-week Picky Eater Project? On a scale of 1 to 10 (1 being no progress; 10 being complete transformation), where do you think you fall so far? Why did you pick the number you picked? What would it take to get to a higher number?

❷ How did your Family Mealtime Mission Statement play into your activities this week?

❸ How closely do you think you followed your rules for "picky-free parenting" this week? Any adjustments that need to be made? How did the kids respond?

❹ What went well?

❺ What was really challenging?

❻ How many times did your child try new foods?

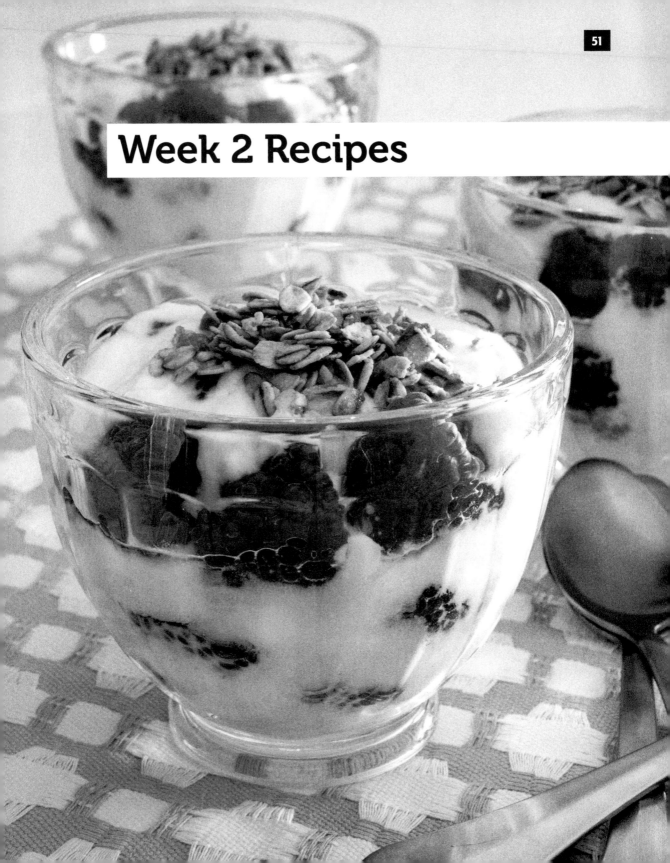

Week 2 Recipes

Parmesan Yogurt Dip With Carrots

Hands-on time: 10 minutes
Total time: 10 minutes
Makes: 2 cups

Greek yogurt is thicker than regular yogurt, which is why Adam Collick, former assistant White House chef, uses it here. We've adapted his recipe but have retained the great flavor and all the benefits. Using Greek yogurt nets a nice thick dip with even more protein than if you use traditional yogurt.

—*Recipe by Adam Collick*

Kitchen Gear
Measuring cup

Sharp knife

Cutting board

Zester or grater

Bowl

Mixing spoon

Ingredients
2 cups plain Greek yogurt

1 small garlic clove, peeled and minced

Juice and grated zest of 1 small lemon

½ cup freshly grated Parmesan cheese

Kosher salt and black pepper to taste

1 bunch (or bag) baby carrots

Instructions
1. Combine the yogurt, garlic, lemon zest and juice, and Parmesan cheese in a bowl and mix well.

2. Add salt and pepper until it tastes the way you like it. Serve with carrots.

Personalize It
Use other vegetables besides (or alongside) carrots, such as

- Celery
- Cucumber
- Cherry tomatoes
- Peppers
- Broccoli
- Cauliflower
- Jicama
- Black olives
- Squash (zucchini/summer squash)

Kids in the Kitchen
- Let your child measure all the ingredients.
- Teach your child how to grate lemon zest and Parmesan cheese.
- Let your child mix and taste test.

Spicy Turkey Chili

Hands-on time: 45 minutes
Total time: 1 hour, 45 minutes
Makes: 12 cups

Chili is pretty great in the winter! It warms you up on the inside.

Kitchen Gear	Ingredients
Can opener	2 teaspoons olive or vegetable oil
Measuring spoons	1 large yellow or purple onion, chopped
Sharp knife	2 bell peppers (any color is fine), seeded and diced
Cutting board	3 garlic cloves, peeled and finely chopped
Measuring cup	1¼ pound ground turkey or chicken
Strainer or colander	2 to 4 tablespoons chili powder
Large heavy-bottomed soup pot with a lid	1½ teaspoon dried oregano
	1 to 2 teaspoons ground cumin
Large spoon	1 teaspoon crushed red pepper flakes (if you like spicy)
Oven mitts	¼ teaspoon cayenne (if you like spicy)
	2 (16-ounce) cans dark red kidney beans, drained and rinsed well with cold water
	1 (16-ounce) can black beans, drained and rinsed well with cold water
	1 (28-ounce) can diced tomatoes, including the juice
	1 (28-ounce) can tomato puree
	1 cup shredded cheddar cheese
	1 cup plain yogurt
	½ cup chopped fresh cilantro leaves
	2 limes, quartered for squeezing

Instructions

1. Place the pot on the stove and turn the heat to medium. When it is hot, add the oil.

2. Add the onion, peppers, and garlic and cook until the onion is very soft, about 20 minutes. Stir from time to time.

3. Add the turkey (or chicken) a little bit at a time, stirring after each addition, until it just starts to turn white. Add the spices and cook, stirring, 5 minutes.

4. Add the beans, tomatoes, and tomato puree and cook covered, stirring occasionally, for 30 minutes.

5. Cook uncovered until thick, about an additional 30 minutes.

6. Serve right away garnished with cheese, yogurt, cilantro leaves, and limes.

Kids in the Kitchen

- Have your child measure each ingredient before adding to the pot.

- Allow your child to stir and mix the ingredients.

- Teach your child how to drain and rinse the beans.

- Show your child how to use a can opener.

Personalize It

- Substitute ground beef for the ground turkey or chicken.

- Vary the beans and substitute chickpeas or white beans.

- Substitute the fresh cilantro with fresh basil leaves.

Sweet Potato Spinach Baby Puree

Hands-on time: 10 minutes
Total time: 25 minutes
Makes: 1 cup

Kitchen Gear

Sharp knife

Cutting board

Measuring cup

Small pot

Handheld blender or masher

Ingredients

1 sweet potato, scrubbed and sliced (The thinner the slices, the faster it will cook.)

¾ cup fresh flat-leaf spinach leaves, finely chopped

Instructions

1. Put the sweet potato slices in the pot, cover with water, and bring to a boil over high heat.

2. Lower the heat to medium, add the spinach, and cook until the sweet potato is tender, about 15 minutes. If necessary, drain off the water.

3. Mash or puree. Set aside to cool to room temperature or cover and refrigerate up to 2 days.

Kids in the Kitchen

- Let your child scrub the sweet potato.

- If using a potato masher, allow your child to mash the mixture.

- If using a food processor, allow your child to press the power buttons.

Personalize It

- Substitute the sweet potato with carrots or butternut squash.

- Substitute the spinach with kale.

Roasted Vegetables

Hands-on time: 20 minutes
Total time: 1 hour, 5 minutes
Makes: 4 to 6 servings

You can eat these hot or cold, alone, or paired with pasta or rice.

Kitchen Gear	**Ingredients**
Measuring cup	1 red onion, diced
Pot holder	1 red bell pepper, seeded and diced
Sharp knife	1 yellow bell pepper, seeded and diced
Cutting board	2 yellow squash, diced
Measuring spoons	2 zucchini, diced
Mixing bowl	4 garlic cloves, peeled, and chopped or minced
Large spoon	1 teaspoon olive oil
Large baking sheet with sides	¼ teaspoon dried thyme
	½ teaspoon kosher salt
	¼ teaspoon black pepper
	2 cups grape or cherry tomatoes

Instructions

1. Turn the oven on and set it to 400 degrees Fahrenheit.

2. Put the onion, bell peppers, squash, zucchini, garlic, olive oil, thyme, salt, and pepper in a bowl and mix well.

3. Pour the vegetables onto a baking sheet, making sure the vegetables are in a single layer. Place the baking sheet in the oven and bake for 25 minutes.

4. Remove the baking sheet from the oven and put it on top of the stove. Add the tomatoes and stir to make sure everything is well mixed.

5. Return to the oven and cook until everything is lightly browned, about 20 minutes. Serve right away or cover and refrigerate up to 2 days.

Roasted Vegetables *(cont)*

Personalize It

Prepare small bowls of the following addtions for before, during, or after cooking:

- Sweet potatoes
- Red potatoes
- Carrots

Kids in the Kitchen

- Show your child how to wash vegetables.
- Have your child mix all of the ingredients together. Quiz your child: How many ingredients did you add? What colors are the ingredients you added?

Layered Yogurt Parfait

Hands-on time: 10 minutes
Total time: 10 minutes
Makes: 4 parfaits

Parfait usually refers to an ice-cream concoction layered in a fancy glass, but it's really a French word that means "perfect." When you try our healthy breakfast version, we think you'll see why!

Kitchen Gear
Sharp knife

Cutting board

Measuring spoon

4 short glasses

Measuring cup

Ingredients
2 cups plain yogurt

2 cups fresh berries or chopped fruit

½ cup homemade or store-bought granola, or a combination of mixed nuts and dried fruit

Instructions
1. Put ¼ cup yogurt in each glass and top with ¼ cup fruit. Repeat once.
2. Top each glass with 2 tablespoons granola and serve right away.

Personalize It
Prepare small bowls of the following additions for before, during, or after cooking:

- Fresh blueberries, strawberries, or raspberries
- Wheat germ
- Nuts (eg, almonds, peanuts, walnuts, pecans)
- Jam (eg, raspberry, blueberry, grape, strawberry, apricot)
- Flavored yogurt (eg, banana, strawberry, vanilla, blueberry)
- Honey

Kids in the Kitchen
- Show your child how to assemble the parfait—use a clear glass so she can see each layer of ingredients.
- Teach your child how to measure ¼ cup of each ingredient.
- Explain to your child that a parfait is typically layered in a pattern—can your child identify the pattern?
- Count how many layers are in the parfait.

Every Kind of Burger (Well, Almost)

Hands-on time: 20 minutes
Total time: 30 minutes
Makes: 4 burgers

A burger will take on the personality of whatever meat you use: chicken or turkey makes a mild burger, lamb makes a very meaty-tasting one, and pork makes a burger that's almost like sausage. Experiment to find out what you like best.

Kitchen Gear	Ingredients
Measuring spoons	1 pound ground chicken, turkey, pork, or lamb
Sharp knife	½ teaspoon kosher salt
Cutting board	¼ teaspoon black pepper (if you like)
Skillet	4 hamburger rolls, sliced in half and toasted (if you like)
Spatula	4 tomato slices
Plate	4 lettuce leaves
	Ketchup, mustard, or special toppings

Instructions

1. Put the raw meat on the cutting board and divide into 4 balls of equal size.

2. Gently press down each ball to form a patty about ¾ to 1 inch thick.

3. Using your thumb, make a ½-inch dent about the size of a quarter in the middle of each side.

4. Sprinkle both sides of the patties with salt (and pepper if you like).

5. Put the skillet on the stove and turn the heat to high. Wait 2 minutes for the pan to heat up and then add the patties to the dry pan.

6. Cook until crusty brown on the outside, about 5 minutes; then flip the patties and cook until crusty brown on the other side, another 5 minutes.

7. Put the bottom half of each roll on a big plate and top each with a burger. Top the burger with a tomato slice and lettuce leaf. Add ketchup, mustard, or other toppings. Then cover with the top of the roll. Serve right away.

Safety Tip

Handle the patties as little as possible, and wash your hands after touching raw meat.

Personalize It

Prepare small bowls of the following additions for after cooking:

- Sliced bell peppers
- Sliced onions
- Cheese slices
- Sliced or mashed avocado

Kids in the Kitchen

- Let your child roll and press the burgers on his own.
- Practice flipping the burgers using a spatula.
- Count how many toppings you can add to your burger.
- See how colorful your toppings are—can you add all the colors of the rainbow?

Energy Bars

Hands-on time: 20 minutes
Total time: 20 minutes
Makes: 16 pieces

These are super fun to make and even better to eat. Serve them for an after-school treat or crumbled on top of yogurt for breakfast.

Kitchen Gear

Measuring cup

Measuring spoons

Wax or parchment paper

Medium-sized bowl

Small bowl

Large spoon

8 × 8 inch pan

Plastic wrap

Dinner knife

Cutting board

Ingredients

½ cup lightly toasted* nuts (one kind or a combination of almonds, walnuts, and pecans)

¾ cup dried fruit (one kind or a combination of raisins, currants, and dried cranberries or chopped dates, prunes, apricots, and peaches)

¾ cup quick-cooking oats

¾ cup crispy-rice cereal

½ cup almond or peanut butter

¼ cup honey or maple syrup

½ teaspoon vanilla extract

Instructions

1. Line the pan with wax or parchment paper and leave enough hanging so you can use it to cover the bars later. (You will need a piece a little more than twice the size of the bottom of the pan.)

2. Put the nuts, dried fruit, oats, rice cereal, and coconut (if using), in the medium-sized bowl and toss well.

3. Put the almond or (peanut butter) and honey in the small bowl and microwave until the butter is softened, about 30 seconds. Stir until smooth. Add the vanilla and stir again until smooth.

4. Pour the almond mixture into the medium-sized bowl and mix with the large spoon until well combined.

5. Dump the mixture into the prepared pan and pat down as hard as you can. You want to make the bars solid (rather than airy). Using the overhanging wax paper, cover the bars completely. Cover with plastic wrap and refrigerate at least 4 hours and up to 1 week.

6. Using the knife, cut into 16 pieces.

*To toast nuts, put them on a small baking sheet in a 350-degree Fahrenheit oven until they are fragrant and look a shade darker, around 5 minutes.

Personalize It

- Add 2 tablespoons unsweetened coconut.
- Add 1 tablespoon flaxseed.

Kids in the Kitchen

- Teach your child how to measure each ingredient.
- Encourage your child to decide which nuts and dried fruit to use.
- Let your child press the energy bars into the pan as hard as she can.

CHAPTER 3

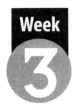

The Little Cook

"This is my invariable advice to people: Learn how to cook— try new recipes, learn from your mistakes, be fearless, and above all have fun."

— Julia Child

Mission
Engage your kids and encourage them to be more excited about trying new foods.

Strategy
Cook together.

Measurement
Kids' ratings of their enjoyment of the cooking experience and how many times they tried a new food.

Prior to the Picky Eater Project, Marlo and Corey rarely involved their kids in cooking and meal preparation. Both working parents and having a thousand other responsibilities and activities to manage, they felt the idea of the extra time and mess that comes with having kids help cook just wasn't worth it. Sally and I, however, felt that involving their kids in cooking would actually prompt the kids to eat healthier foods and not refuse so much of the food that Marlo and Corey made, so Marlo and Corey agreed to give it a try. After all, they were getting a little bit sick of forcing their kids to eat their vegetables.

In pediatrics, we often advise parents and our patients of the easy-to-remember 5-2-1-0 concept for good health. This translates into eating vegetables and fruits at least 5 times per day, spending less than 2 hours on noneducational screen time activities (children older than 2 years), being physically active at least 60 minutes per day, and aiming for 0 sugary drinks such as sodas and juice. Parents are aware of a big disconnect in what is recommended versus reality, and it can cause a lot of anxiety. While the natural response might be to push your kids to eat more healthy food and remind them to eat less junk food, we know this doesn't work most of the time. What we have found does work is gentle and strategic nudges. And the most important nudge of all is introducing kids to the kitchen and teaching them how to cook.

Recognizing the importance of teaching kids to cook, we recommend starting out the Picky Eater Project with kids in the kitchen from day 1. In many cases, having a chance to cook is what is most exciting about the whole project. In fact, when we were working with Brooke and Hunter, when Brooke learned about the project, she squealed, "You mean I get to learn how to cook!" and ran to the kitchen drawer to get out her apron.

When kids are involved in helping to choose and make the food they are expected to eat, they are much more likely to try it. During week 3, Marlo and Corey experienced this firsthand as Brooke, who would often be the first to reject a new food, experimented with a variety of recipes and even when they didn't turn out so great tried them anyway, prompting Marlo to reflect: "No way would she have tried that if I had made it and it turned out that way!" Corey added that having Hunter help put the salt, pepper, and barbeque sauce on grilled chicken has transformed that meal since now Hunter will actually try the chicken he helped season.

Preschool Picky Eater Project

We noticed a similar reaction to cooking with another family that Sally worked with in helping picky 4-year-old twins to become a little more adventurous. Christine and her husband, Fran, considered one twin, Andrew, the picky one. He turned his nose up at everything, while his brother, Nathaniel, tried more foods. Christine and Fran decided to make small changes such as inviting the twins to help pick out and make dinners. A transformation occurred quickly! The twins made their own pizzas and piled on kale and broccoli among a smorgasbord of veggies to choose from, which they ate. But we know it is unrealistic for 2 working parents to cook with two 4-year-olds on a daily basis, and it is unrealistic for 4-year-olds to always be eager to eat vegetables. Case in point, later that same week, Christine, in a rush to get dinner on the table, made broccoli pizzas without the help of the boys. When Andrew looked at his plate, his eyes filled with tears. "I don't want this," he said. "I want cheese and pepperoni." After Christine reinforced the "this is dinner" message, he ate the raw vegetables on his plate except for the red pepper. Then he ate the pizza around the broccoli. However, he didn't ask for something else, which was a great victory. As the takeaway, Christine observed that the interactive cooking process was a buffer against the new, giving the boys time to accept, anticipate, and even appreciate what they were about to eat, even if it's not all the time.

Teaching kids to be involved in cooking in an age-appropriate way not only serves the important purpose of nudging the kids toward healthier eating but also offers a lot of other equally important benefits. Cooking teaches kids academic skills—math (measuring ingredients), chemistry (fermentation, emulsification), and reading and following instructions (recipes)—as well as social skills (working together to achieve a shared goal) and an important life skill (being able to throw together a balanced meal). As Guy Fieri, a chef on Food Network notes: "Cooking with kids is not just about ingredients, recipes, and cooking. It's about harnessing imagination, empowerment, and creativity."

Getting the kids in the kitchen does not need to be elaborate or time-consuming. In fact, Marlo and Corey found that work commitments sidelined some of their best plans for cooking together as a family. Despite the schedule, they still were able to squeeze in supervising Brooke and Hunter making pancakes on Sunday. We highlight their experience within our 5-step recipe for success in the Teaching Kids to Cook section as a strategy to prevent or undo picky eating.

Teaching Kids to Cook: A 5-Star Recipe

❶ Invite kids in the kitchen early and often. We started Brooke and Hunter cooking with their parents from the first week of the Picky Eater Project because we know that when kids participate in picking out and preparing a food, they are much more likely to eat it. By involving them—even if it is just every now and then—you will help them muster the courage to taste a new food. Of course, we realize having kids in the kitchen can be a bit messy at first and not much of a time-saver; in fact, quite the opposite, at least with younger kids. But if you take the time early on to get them involved, teach them to pick up after themselves, and engage them in the whole process of putting a meal on the table—including planning, preparing, setting the table, and cleaning up—you *will* eventually save time. In fact, one day, when old enough, they might even cook for you!

Most important, you will help them broaden their taste preferences and teach them how to prepare healthy foods (which will serve them very well down the road when they have to take care of themselves) as well as spend some quality family time together and catch up on what's going on in their lives. In Table 3.1, we offer ideas on how you can involve kids of every age in the kitchen.

Table 3.1. Kids Can Help Cook at Any Age

Age/Stage	Kitchen Tasks (All tasks should be supervised by an adult.)
Toddler (1–3 years)	• Sift dry contents. • Stir ingredients. • "Paint" pans/vegetables/chicken with oil with pastry brush. • Practice play dough with real dough and cookie cutters. • Pick fresh herbs from garden/windowsill. • Help arrange foods into interesting shapes and designs.
Preschool (4–5 years)	• Rinse produce. • Measure dry ingredients. • Mix simple ingredients. • Cut soft fruits or vegetables with a dull knife or dough scraper. • Push down on the blender/food processor button. • Season foods with salt/pepper/herbs. • Grease pan.
School (6–12 years)	• Read recipe. • Peel vegetables. • Crack egg. • Prep lettuce for salad. • Measure and mix dry and wet ingredients. • Open cans.
Teen (13–17 years)	• Follow a simple recipe. • Boil pasta. • Chop vegetables. • Plan balanced meals.

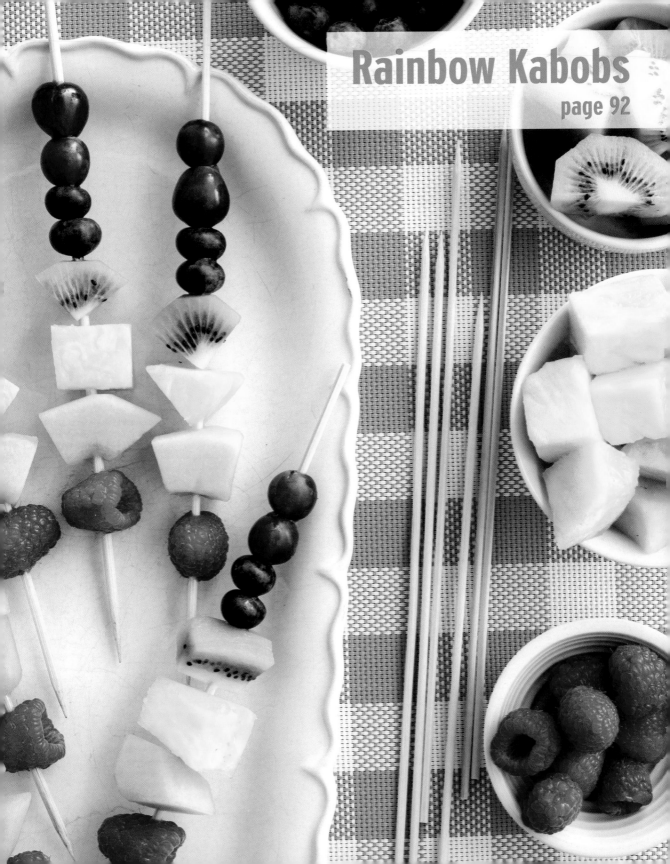

Rainbow Kabobs
page 92

Vietnamese Chicken Noodle Soup
page 99

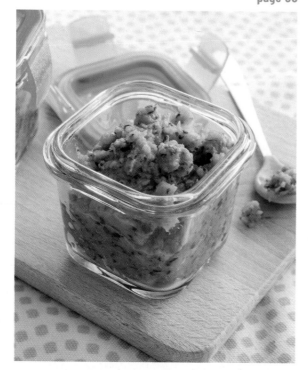

Mixed-up Eggs and Spinach
page 27

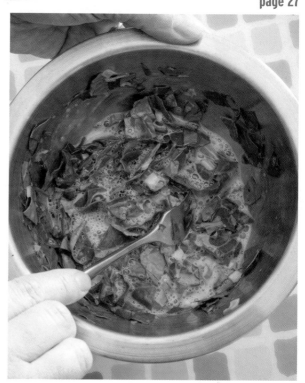

Sweet Potato Spinach Baby Puree
page 56

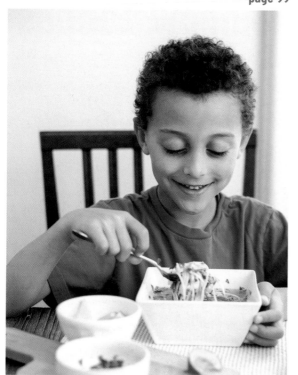

Chicken Fingers
page 25

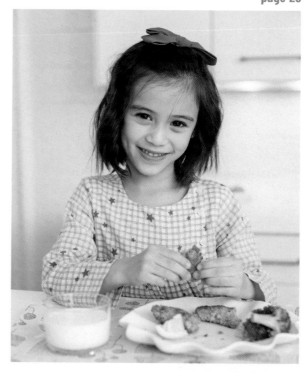

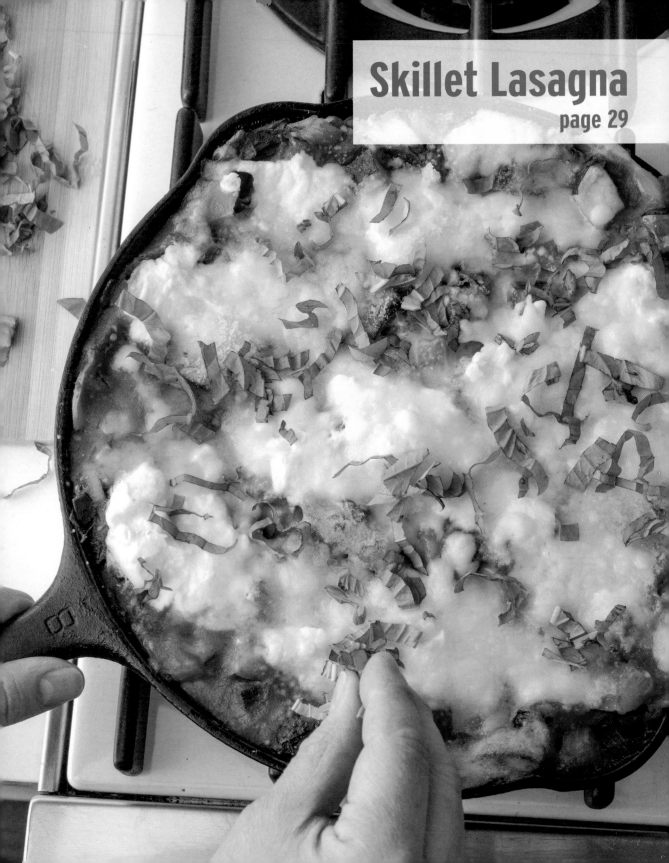

Basic Mix-and-Match Smoothie

page 81

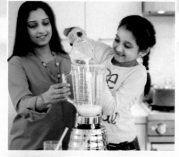

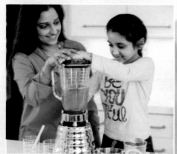

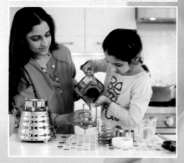

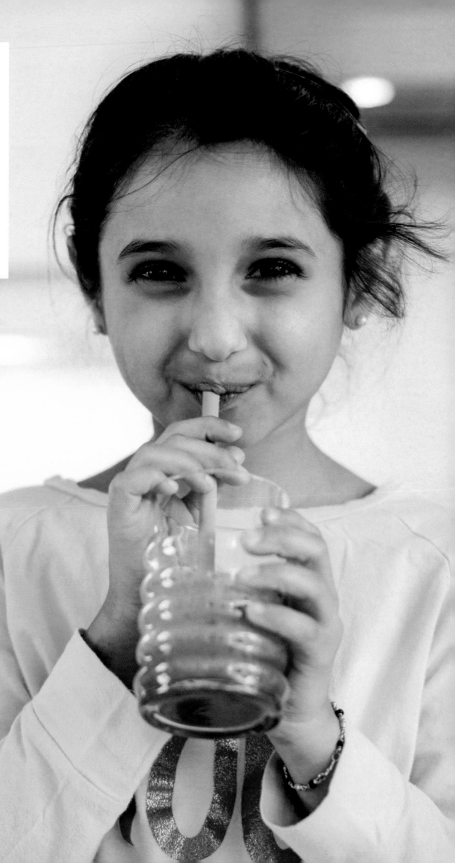

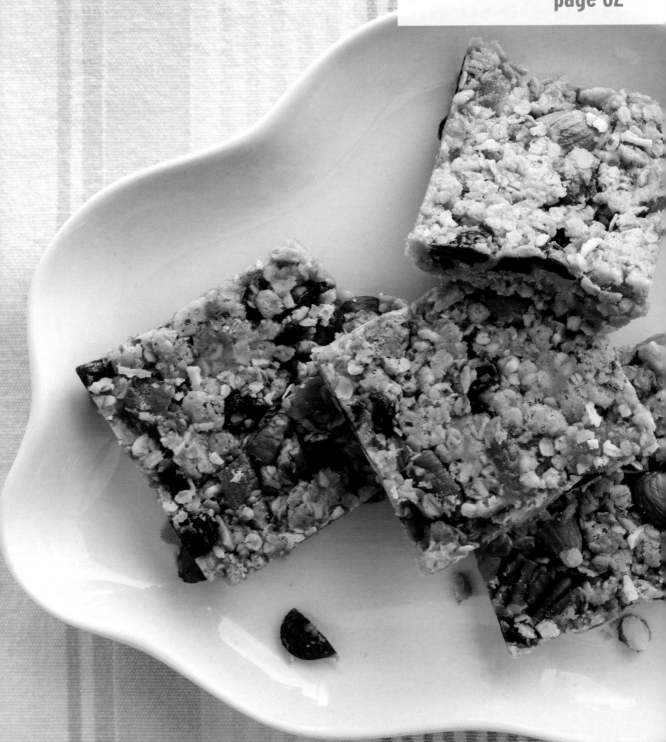

Energy Bars
page 62

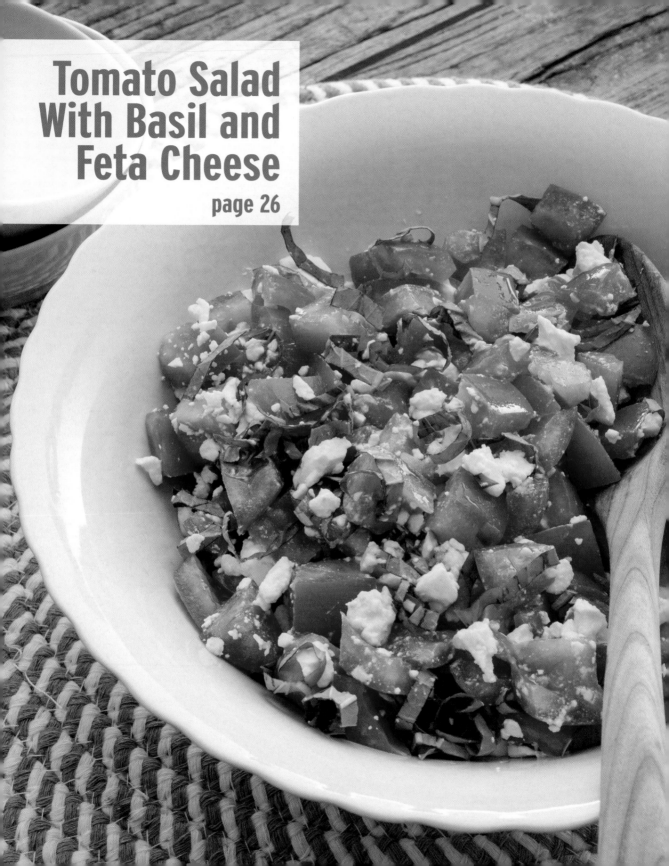

Tomato Salad With Basil and Feta Cheese

page 26

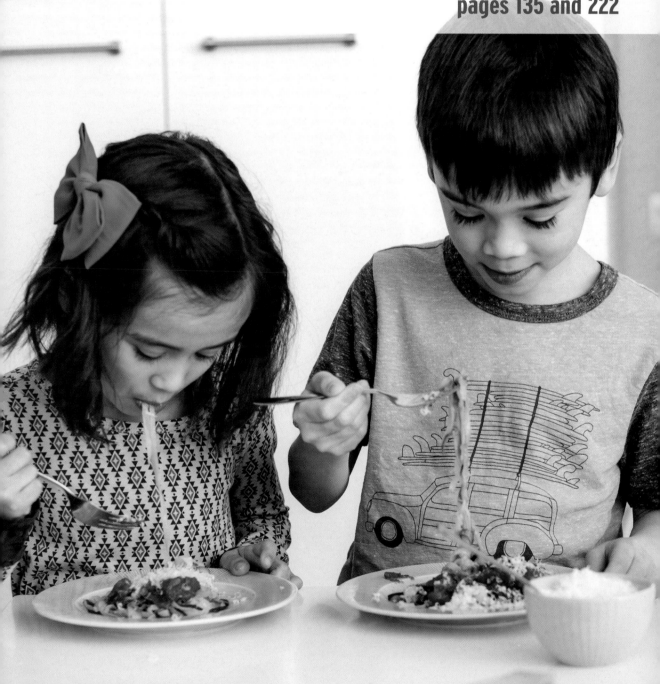

Zucchini Pasta With World's Quickest Tomato Sauce

pages 135 and 222

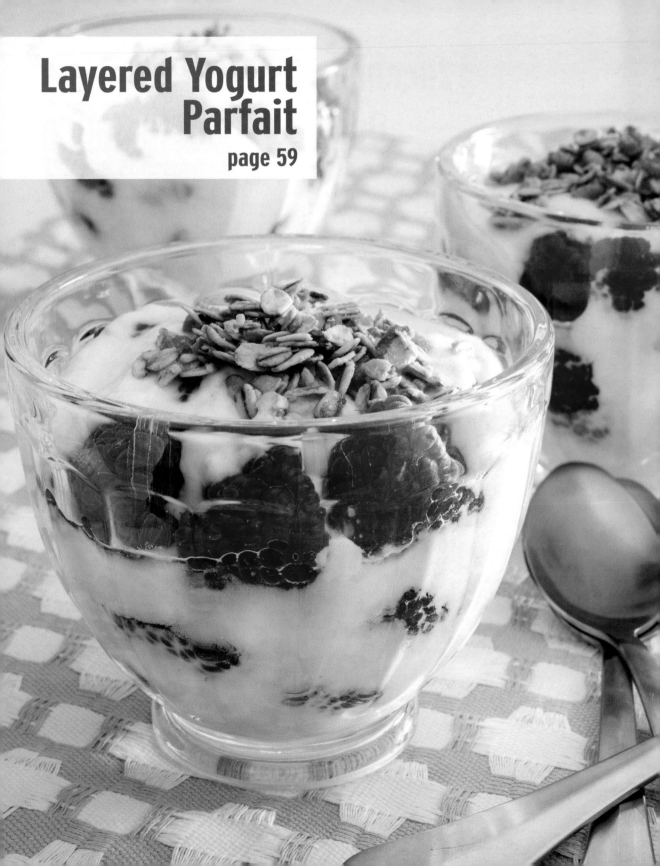

Layered Yogurt
Parfait
page 59

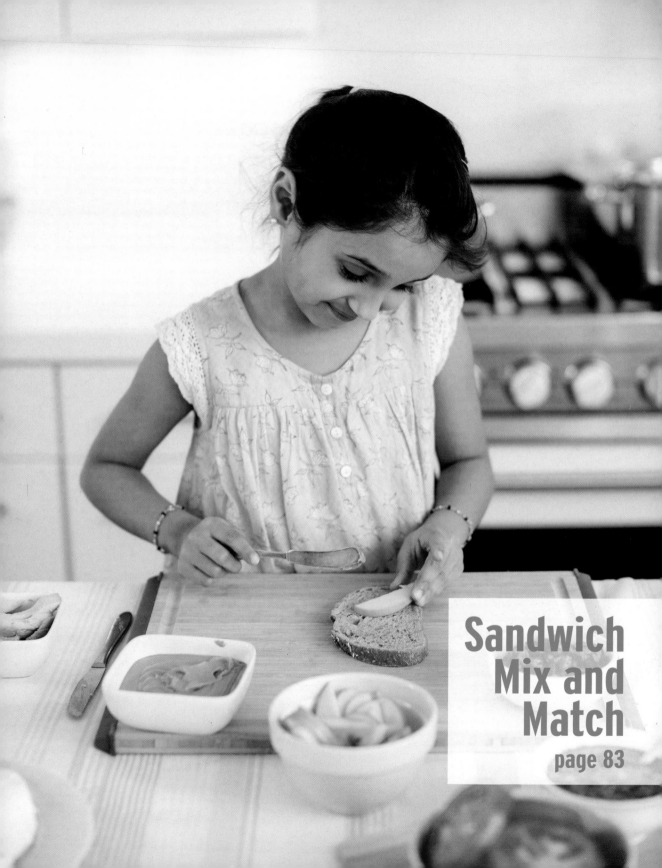

Sandwich
Mix and
Match
page 83

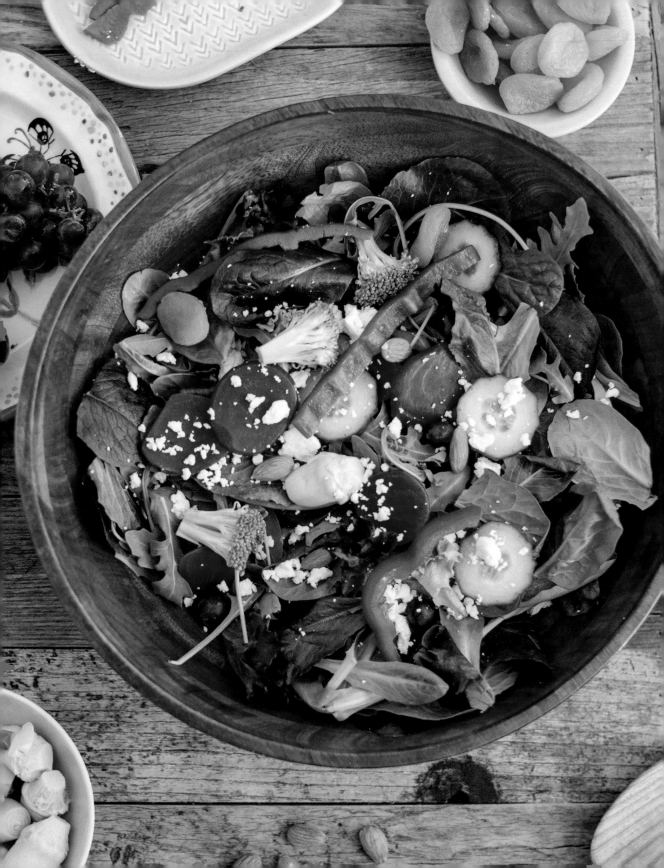

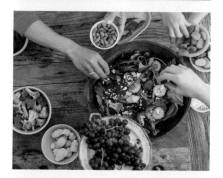

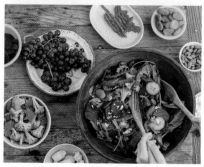

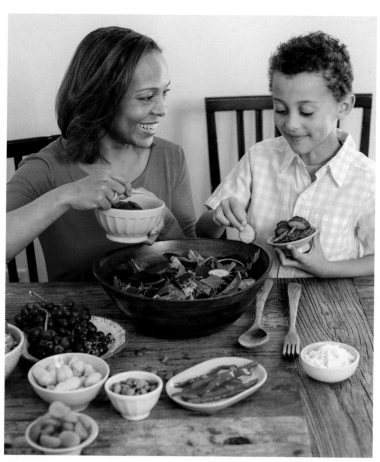

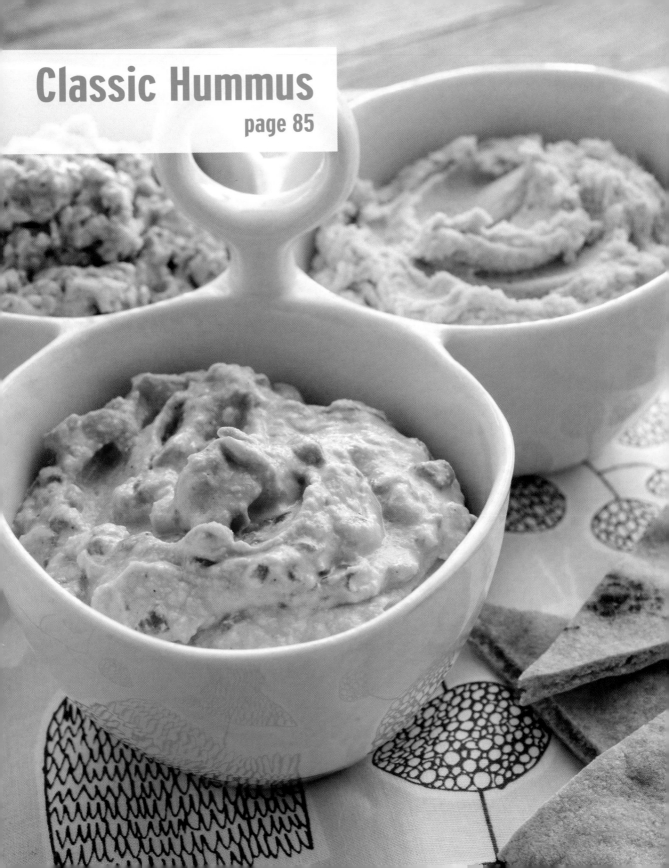

Classic Hummus
page 85

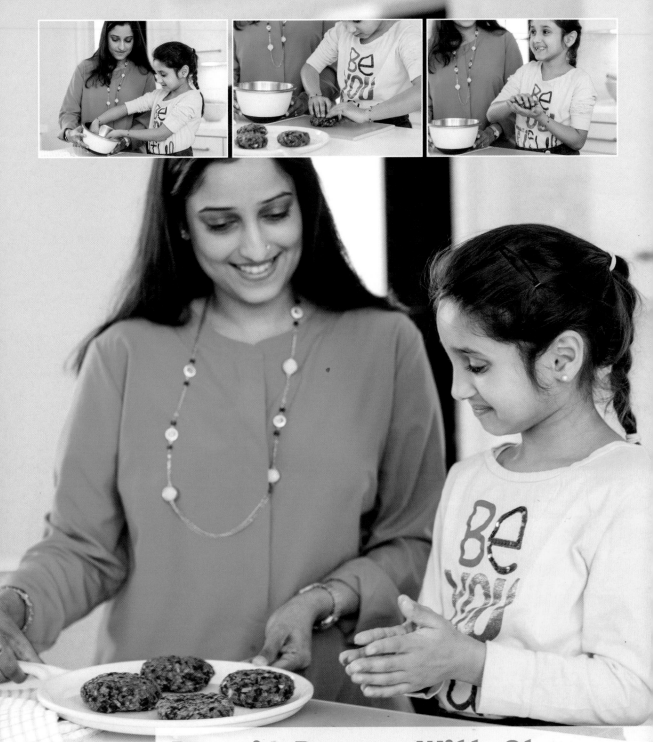

Beanie Burger With Cheese
page 93

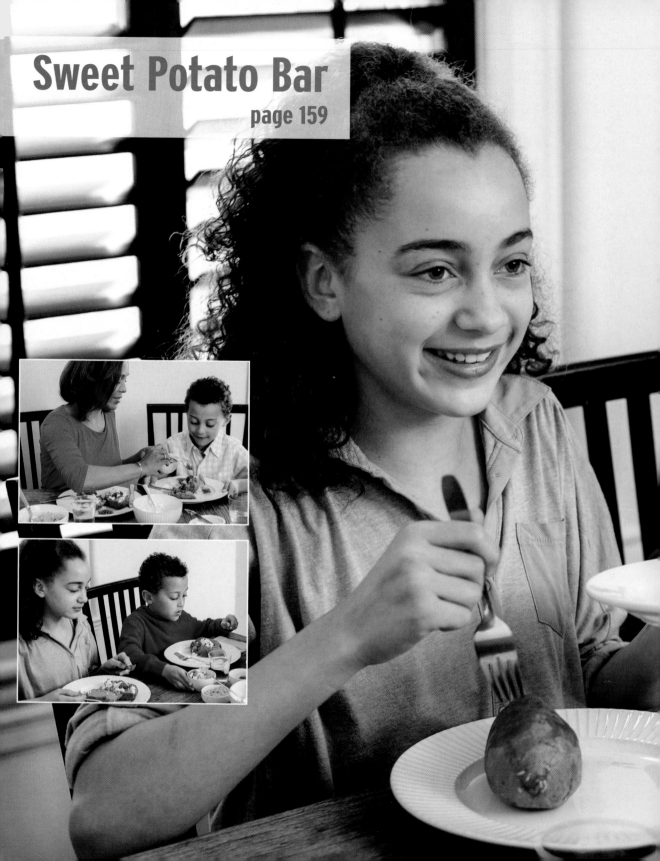

Sweet Potato Bar

page 159

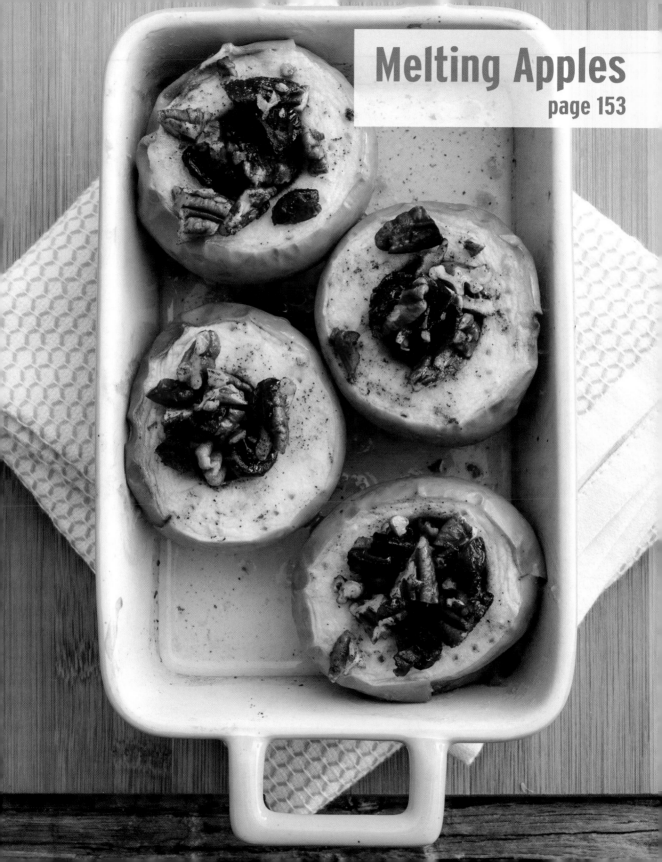

Melting Apples
page 153

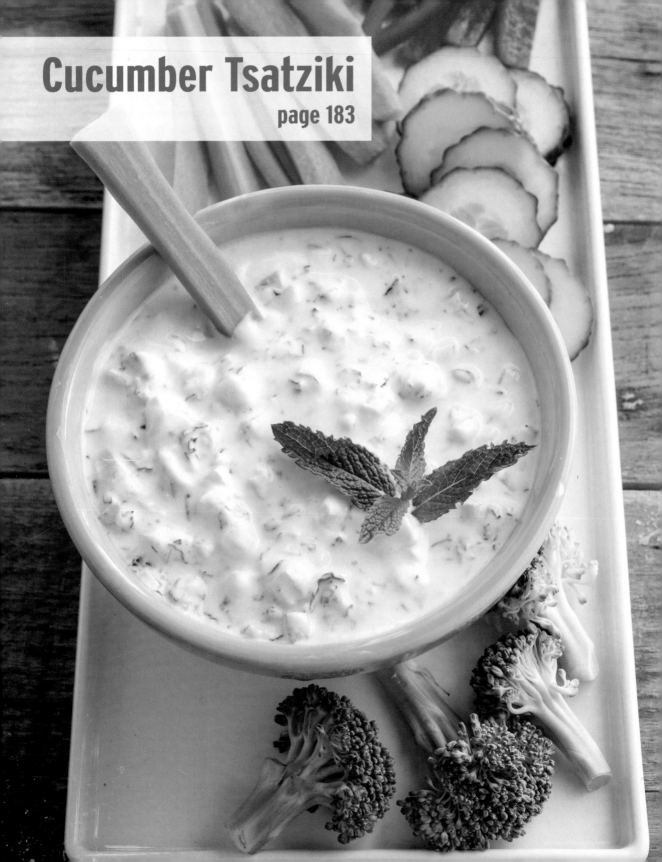

Cucumber Tsatziki
page 183

❷ **Choose the recipe wisely.** Putting some thought into what foods you are choosing to cook is vital for a successful cooking experience. With Brooke and Hunter we chose corn pancakes for a few reasons. First, we knew they already liked pancakes, and might also find they like corn by pairing it with a favorite food. Second, one of Brooke's goals of the project was to practice flipping pancakes, so we knew she'd be motivated. Third, the recipe is simple with just a few ingredients and easy-to-follow instructions—key features for novice cooks. Finally, corn pancakes smell good, look good, and taste *really* good—all factors that increase the odds kids will actually be willing to try them. If you'd like to try this for yourself with your own kids, see our Double Corn Cakes With Fresh Corn recipe on page 97.

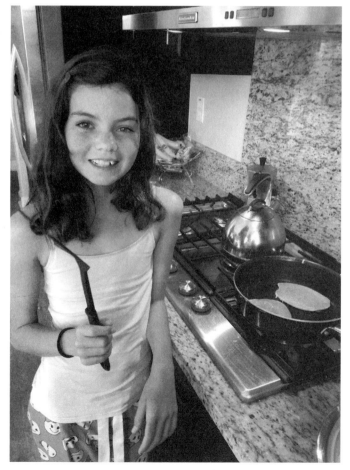

One way to increase the odds that your child will be willing to try a new food is through bridging—choosing a recipe that is very similar in taste or texture to a food your child already enjoys. For example, if your child loves breaded chicken nuggets and you'd like your child to be more accepting of fish, you might try a recipe with fish nuggets. Once that is well accepted, you might next transition to a lightly breaded fish and ultimately to the healthier grilled fish.

Read through the entire recipe before you start to be sure you understand all the instructions, have all the ingredients, and have a plan for how your child might best help you prepare the dish. Follow the recipe steps and review the ingredient list a few times to make sure you've used everything in the correct order and amount.

❸ **Learn basic cooking methods.** Kids are sensitive to tastes and textures when deciding whether to try a food. This means a child who might outright reject raw broccoli with ranch dip may be more than happy to eat homemade broccoli cheddar soup, or say no to roasted chicken but love barbeque chicken. The only way to find this out is to offer new foods in different ways, using different food combinations and cooking methods. Of course, time and energy to spend in the kitchen—much less supervising your kids spending time in the kitchen—is limited. Check Sally's Top 10 Tips for Beginner Chefs (Box 3.1) and Table 3.2 for recipes by meal type.

Box 3.1. Sally's Top 10 Tips for Beginner Chefs

Learning to cook may seem overwhelming at first, but it doesn't need to be! Even the most admired chefs had to learn to cook at some point, with many "interesting" outcomes. If you or your kids are just getting started in the kitchen, or if you consider yourself to be a little more seasoned, these few ideas might help you have a more fun and successful cooking experience.

❶ Keep a full pantry (eg, spices, oils, vinegars, canned tomatoes, beans). See Box 2.1, The Picky Eater Project Pantry Guide, on page 39.

❷ Keep everything safe: wear closed-toed shoes, keep knives away from edges, use pot holders, and focus on each cooking step in a recipe you and your child are working on together.

❸ Taste as you go. Even if a dish is new to you, what matters most is that YOU like what you are eating. Experiment with a little more of this herb or seasoning and little less of that one as you go to make the dish taste just right for you.

❹ Read the recipe from beginning to end *before you start*!

❺ Be OK with making mistakes!

❻ Don't worry too much about making a mess.

❼ But clean as you go.

❽ Take your time.

❾ Be OK if family doesn't like something, but be sure they're respectful (in other words, no "ewwws").

❿ Have fun!

WHAT'S YOUR STORY 🍎❓

- Have you ever rallied your kids to help with the cooking? If not, why not? If so, how did it go?

- What is one tip from this chapter that sticks out to you the most? Up your cooking IQ by making a few small changes based on that tip this week.

Table 3.2. Meal Ideas

Eating regular, balanced meals helps set the stage for healthy eating patterns. Incorporating a balanced breakfast, lunch, and dinner helps kids get needed nutrients as well as provides a steady source of energy to optimize academic performance, physical activity, and mood. This balanced eating plan also offers many opportunities to nudge kids toward more open-minded meal habits. Tips for taking advantage of various meals and snacks to undo picky eating preferences are included here.

Meal Type	The Lowdown	Recipe
Breakfast	Kids may wake up in the morning very hungry. But time is also very limited for most families. Use breakfast as an opportunity to get in a quick meal and the first serving of fruit for the day.	Basic Mix-and-Match Smoothie (For recipe, see page 81.)
Lunch	Encourage your kids to make their own lunch, offering them just the following guidance for what must be in there: Include a grain, protein, fruit, vegetable, and dairy product.	Sandwich Mix and Match (See page 83.)
Dips and spreads	Dips are oftentimes a kid favorite and offer a great way to introduce new vegetables. When the kids are at their hungriest, set out a veggie tray with one or more sampling dips. A hungry child will eat!	Classic Hummus (See page 85.)
Soups	A warm soup on a cold night is a crowd-pleaser and also a great way to introduce your kids to new vegetables. For kids who are texture sensitive, start with a broth and then try some of our creamy vegetable soups before offering full-textured soups like minestrone.	(Almost) Any Vegetable Soup (See page 87.)
Salads	Many kids are quick to refuse all things green, but it doesn't have to be that way! Try growing a small garden (lettuce is very easy to grow in abundance) and see if the kids may be willing to try some of the food they helped grow.	The Salad (See page 89.)

Table 3.2 *(cont)*

Meal Type	The Lowdown	Recipe
Snacks	Snacks can be an important part of a healthy, balanced eating plan but too often they include heavily processed, sugary, or salty foods. Set your kids up for success by making available vegetables, fruits, and portion-controlled whole grains, proteins, or dairy for snacks.	Rainbow Kabobs (See page 92.)
Dinner	The best dinners include a good source of whole grain, protein, vegetable, and fruit. If you incorporate these ingredients into most family dinners, your kids will start to learn what balanced looks like, even if they don't eat in a balanced way at first. Your modeling pays off over time!	Beanie Burger With Cheese *(on whole-grain bread with lettuce, tomato, and orange slices)* (See page 93.)
Vegetables	Before calling a vegetable hopeless, try offering it raw, steamed, or roasted to see if a different texture may be more acceptable to your child. For example, many times a child who can't stand steamed broccoli is happy to eat it roasted or raw with ranch dip.	Oven-Roasted Broccoli (See page 95.)
Desserts	Consider desserts an occasional food. When having them (we suggest no more than 2–3 times per week unless they are fruit without added sugars), avoid keeping leftovers in the house or making a big deal out of them. We advise caution in using desserts as a reward, especially in exchange for eating vegetables and other healthy foods. This creates a mind-set that desserts are much more delicious and healthy foods are so undesirable a child has to be bribed to eat them.	Banana-Peach Frozen Yogurt (See page 96.)

WHAT'S YOUR STORY ?

Ready to put some of this advice to good use? Together with your kids, pick one recipe from Table 3.2 on page 73, purchase any ingredients you don't already have, and together make the recipe. Pay attention to if your kids try any new foods while they are helping make the meal and if they ate the food in the end. What else did you observe?

❹ Engage all of your senses, especially taste. Cooking engages all of the senses—touch, smell, sights, sounds, and, most especially, taste. The main predictor of whether a child will eat a new food is the perception or experience of it tasting good. It can take a child up to 15 to 20 times to train the taste buds to like a particular food. The mere experience of tasting the food will make it more likely the child will like the food down the road, even if the child ends up spitting it out. The taste buds are on the tongue and the benefit comes from merely activating those taste buds. Following a recipe isn't enough to know if it is going to turn out right for your family. You'll need to taste the dishes as they're cooking to test if they taste just right or if you need a little bit more of something to make the flavor pop. More herbs, lemon, garlic, or pepper? The only way you'll know is if you taste it. Check out our seasoning taste bud experiment (Try It Out: A Taste Bud Explosion).

❺ Have fun with it. Try substituting ingredients based on what your kids feel like. Let them choose the most outrageous concoctions and see how it turns out. Go on a pretend "trip around the world" by learning about various countries and then prepare traditional meals from some of those countries (Box 3.2 has ideas). Or, once a month, make dinner a festive celebration by having your kids decorate and be responsible for serving the hors d'oeuvres of their choice. You might even consider picking up a kid's apron and chef hat to make cooking feel even more fun.

While we are always eager to nudge kids toward healthier choices, if it turns out that kids aren't that interested in learning to cook, that's OK too. As chef Todd English said, "Like anything, you don't force kids to cook. It just becomes part of life—have them be around it, keep them informed—talk about it. I try to relay my passion for it in these ways. The second you try to force anything on your own kid[s], they rebel."

TRY IT OUT

A Taste Bud Explosion

One of the most important skills you can develop as a cook is learning to taste food. That means you taste a dish before you serve it, to figure out if it needs anything—even if you've already added all the ingredients listed in the recipe. You have your own preferences and different ingredients will require different adjustments. You'll want to learn how to season food so that it tastes as good to you as it could possibly taste. To learn a little bit about some of the main seasoning elements, gather your kids in the kitchen and try this together:

Kitchen Gear

Vegetable peeler

Medium-sized pot with lid

Sharp knife (adult needed)

Colander

Ingredients

1 potato, scrubbed or peeled, and cubed

Kosher salt

1 lemon, cut in half

Black pepper

Other seasonings, including salsa, ground cinnamon, pesto, any kind of vinegar, cayenne pepper, curry powder, fresh garlic, hot sauce, grated lemon zest and/or whatever else you like (or would like to try).

Instructions

Put the cubed potato pieces in the pot and fill it halfway with cold water. Put it on the stove, turn the heat to high and bring the water to a boil. You'll know the water is boiling when you see bubbles breaking all over the surface.

Lower the heat to medium and cook until the potato is tender, about 15 minutes.

Put the colander in the sink. Pour the potatoes into the colander and set them aside until cooled, about 20 minutes.

Take a cube of potato and eat it plain. What does it taste like?

- Sprinkle a little salt on a cube and taste it.

- Squeeze a little lemon juice on a cube and taste it.

- Grind or shake a little pepper on a cube and taste it.

- Now combine the seasonings and figure out what your perfect balance is: How much salt? How much lemon? How much pepper?

- Experiment with the additional seasonings to see what you like best.

Reproduced with permission from Sally Sampson. Original source: Sampson S. *ChopChop: The Kids' Guide to Cooking Real Food with Your Family.* New York, NY: Simon & Schuster; 2013.

Box 3.2. A Trip Around the World (From the Comfort of Your Own Kitchen)

A great way to pique your kids' interest in trying interesting foods, which otherwise might be rejected, is through the excitement of an exotic excursion—from the comfort of your own kitchen! Together as a family, pick a country all of you would like to learn more about. Assign everyone something to research (eg, ethnic cuisine, style of dress, traditions, arts, cultural values) and be prepared to share your exciting findings at the Sunday dinner. As part of the adventure, prepare a traditional recipe from that country.

Here's an example.

- Country of the month: Vietnam

- Continent: Asia

- Capital: Hanoi

- Population: approximately 90 million

Traditional meal philosophy. Application of the principles of yin and yang to provide balance for meals, especially in pairing hot and cold, such as spicy ("hot") with sourness ("cool").

Commonly eaten foods. Steamed long-grain white rice is a staple at nearly every meal. In general, rice is used to make other common ingredients such as rice noodles (eg, pho, vermicelli), rice paper wrappers, wine, and rice vinegar. Fruits, vegetables, fish sauce (nuoc mam), shrimp pasta, dipping sauce (*nuoc chom*), and an abundance of fresh herbs (eg, lemongrass, ginger, mint, coriander, lime, Thai basil) are also very common.

Traditional dishes. Pho (noodle soup), *goi cuon* (spring rolls), and *bánh mì* (bread, but often refers to baguette sandwich filled with meats and an abundance of Vietnamese herbs and vegetables).

Most meals are very healthy and contain a balance of 5.

- Tastes: spicy, sour, bitter, salty, and sweet

- Types of nutrients: carbohydrate, water or liquid, mineral elements, protein, and fat

- Colors: white, green, yellow, red, and black

- Senses: food arrangement (eyes), sounds (crisp), spices and herbs (taste), herbs (smell), finger foods (touching)

Now create your own Vietnamese culinary adventure with our Vietnamese Chicken Noodle Soup recipe on page 99!

YOUR PICKY EATER PROJECT—WEEK 3

The Little Cook

Project To-dos Checklist

☐ Together with your kids, pick a recipe you'd like to try. Keep in mind your overall goals of this 6-week Picky Eater Project and your child's preferences. Consider the recipes in this book, *ChopChop: The Kids' Guide to Cooking Real Food with Your Family,* or *ChopChop* magazine for inspiration.

How did it go?

☐ Try the seasoning experiment (see Try It Out: A Taste Bud Explosion on page 76).

What happened?

☐ Involve your kids in the weekly goal-setting process. Maybe they will want to choose from one of the following goals or brainstorm an idea of their own:

- Make a single snack recipe.
- Pick a night you'll make dinner with a parent or another adult every week.
- Pack your own lunch.
- Volunteer to make breakfast on the weekend.
- Invite a friend over to cook with you.

Project Check-in

❶ Reflect back on the last 3 weeks. What change sticks out the most for you? What one change were you hoping for that you haven't seen yet? What ideas do you have that might help you get closer to that change?

❷ How well did you practice your "picky-free parenting" rules this week?

❸ What was the greatest challenge in cooking with your kids? What was the greatest reward?

❹ On a scale of 1 to 10 (1 being the least enjoyable; 10 being the most), how enjoyable was this week for you? Ask your kids the same question. How did it turn out? What worked well? What could be better next time?

❺ How many times did your children try new foods?

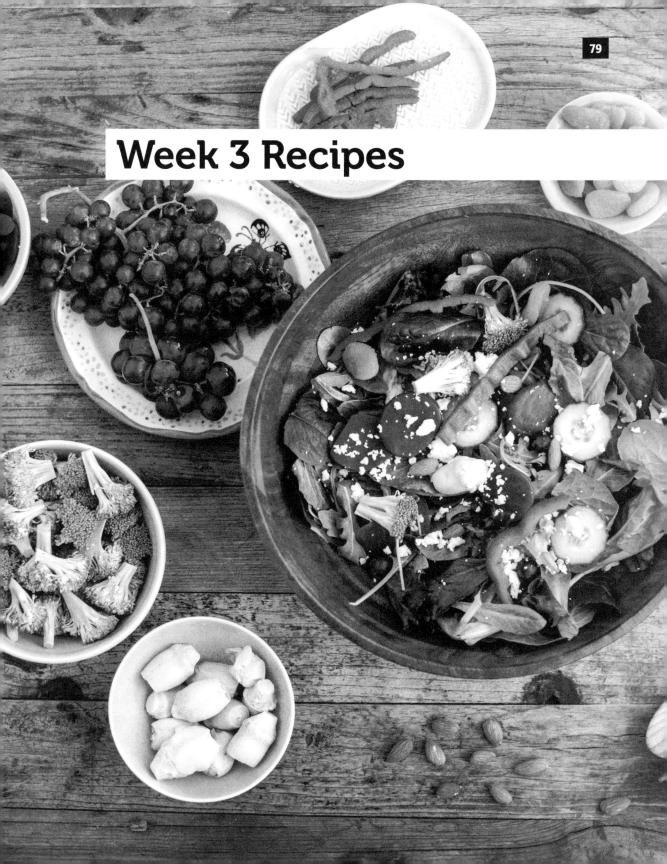

Week 3 Recipes

Basic Mix-and-Match Smoothie

Hands-on time: 10 minutes
Total time: 10 minutes
Makes: 2 servings

Why not enjoy a cool, fruity smoothie for breakfast! It's also great for snack time or at lunch. Just give it a shake before drinking to make sure all the ingredients are blended. Below is a chart for mixing and matching. Certain fruits are particularly good with other fruits and with other ingredients, too. But don't take our word for it: experiment to your heart's delight!

Kitchen Gear

Measuring cup

Measuring spoons

Sharp knife

Cutting board

Blender

Ingredients

Fruit, Fresh or Frozen	Liquid	Extras	If You Like...
1 cup (Mix and match.)	1 cup	1–2 tablespoons	A handful kale or spinach
Peaches	½ cup plain yogurt plus ½ cup water	Almonds, walnuts, or pecans	2 ice cubes
Berries			A dash of ground cinnamon or vanilla extract
Apples	Or Low-fat milk	Or Wheat germ	
Oranges			
Banana	Or Non-dairy milk, such as soy, almond, coconut or flax milk	Or Ground flaxseed	
Pineapple		Or Peanut or almond butter	1 teaspoon honey or real maple syrup
Mango			
	Or Rice milk or coconut water		

Basic Mix-and-Match Smoothie *(cont)*

Instructions

1. Pour the liquid ingredients in the blender; then add the desired cut-up fruit (peel or seed it if you need to), as well as the extras.

2. Secure the blender top on tightly. Turn the blender to medium and blend until the mixture is smooth, about 2 minutes.

3. Divide the smoothie between the 2 cups and scrape out the rest with a spoon.

4. Serve right away or cover and refrigerate up to 4 hours.

Personalize It

- Have your kids choose whichever ingredients they'd like in their smoothie!

- Challenge your child to add as many ingredients as she can.

- Have your child count how many ingredients she used.

Kids in the Kitchen

- Taste different fruits, nuts, and other add-ins before adding.

- Play a prediction game: Can you guess what color the smoothie will be after blending?

- Let your children press the buttons on the blender—they love having this control!

- Teach your child how to measure ingredients.

- Have your child count ice cubes.

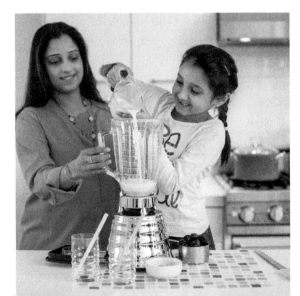

Sandwich Mix and Match

Hands-on time: 20 minutes
Total time: 1 hour, 5 minutes
Makes: 4 to 6 servings

Sure, lettuce and tomato are great, but a wide world of possibility for sandwiches is out there! Don't limit yourself to the usual, or even to what we suggest here. As long as you've got a good balance of protein and vegetables, textures and tastes, and a whole lot of colors, you're going to have a sandwich that satisfies your mouth's flavor cravings and your body's energy requirements.

Base (Pick 1.)	Protein (Pick 1.)	Vegetable (Pick 2 or 3.)	Fruit (Pick 1.)	Condiments and Dips
Whole-wheat bread or toast	Chicken salad	Shredded carrots or purple cabbage	Sliced pears	Pesto
Wrap	Egg salad or sliced boiled eggs	Greens, including romaine lettuce, mesclun, or spinach	Sliced grapes	Beet or Cucumber Tsatziki (For recipe, see Chapter 6, page 183.)
Multigrain bagel	Smoked ham	Sliced radishes	Sliced pineapple	Dijon mustard
Tortilla	Turkey	Avocado	Dried cranberries	Hummus
Whole-wheat English muffin	Tuna salad or sardines	Sliced tomato	Sliced apples	Guacamole
Pita	Hummus	Ratatouille or Roasted Vegetables (For recipe, see Chapter 2, page 57.)	Fresh peaches	Sliced pickles
Multigrain roll	Cheese	Sprouts	Raisins	Capers
Whole-wheat hamburger or hot dog bun	Peanut butter	Sliced cucumbers	Banana	Apple butter

Personalize It

Fifteen sandwiches to spark your imagination and taste buds!

1. Chicken and Brie cheese with apple slices and apple butter

2. Smoked turkey and sliced avocado with shredded carrots

3. Smoked ham and cheddar cheese with cucumber slices and mango chutney or apple butter

4. Smoked ham with cucumber slices, pineapple slices, and mustard

5. Tuna salad with sprouts, sliced radishes, and sliced grapes

Sandwich Mix and Match *(cont)*

6. Sardines with mashed avocado, cucumber slices, and tomato slices

7. Egg salad or sliced egg with sprouts and capers

8. Egg salad or sliced egg with beet or Cucumber Tsatziki (For recipe, see Chapter 6, page 183.)

9. Feta cheese and Roasted Vegetables with shredded carrots (For recipe, see page 57.)

10. Cheddar cheese and mashed avocado with tomato and pickles

11. Mozzarella cheese with tomato slices and pesto

12. Brie with spinach leaves and sliced peaches

13. Hummus and Roasted Vegetables (For recipe, see Chapter 2, page 57.)

14. Hummus with cucumber slices and tomato slices

15. Peanut butter with apple slices, banana slices, and raisins

Tip!

Who needs bread? A large lettuce leaf makes a great sandwich wrap. Just be sure to use at least one filling that will hold everything together, such as hummus or Guacamole (for recipe, see Chapter 6, page 184); then lay the rest of the ingredients on top, roll up your leaf nice and tight, and munch away.

Hate soggy sandwiches? Everybody does. Here's how you can avoid sogginess.

- Put a single layer of meat or cheese on each slice of bread, spread the condiments on those, and then stuff the vegetables and rest of the filling in the middle. The meat or cheese protects the bread from the soggy elements.

- Before you add tomatoes, cucumbers, pickles, or other drippy ingredients to your sandwich, blot them on a paper towel.

- Pack your sandwich in parts, and assemble it at lunchtime. You'll need a plastic container with a lid: start with the bread on the bottom, then layer your sandwich ingredients between pieces of waxed paper, and finish with a small container of any wet ingredients, such as mustard or hummus. Or assemble most of your sandwich, and just leave out anything damp or wet, such as tomatoes or pickles, which you can pack separately and add later. Don't forget a butter knife for spreading!

Kids in the Kitchen

- Let your child taste test ingredients before adding.

- Have your child assemble the sandwich.

- Challenge him to create a pattern with the ingredients.

- Ask him how many ingredients he can add to his sandwich.

Classic Hummus

Hands-on time: 15 minutes
Total time: 15 minutes
Makes: 1½ cups

Here's a bean dip you're probably familiar with: hummus, the classic Middle Eastern dip of chickpeas, tahini (sesame paste), garlic, and lemon juice. Once you start making it yourself, you will be really surprised that anyone buys it in a container! We love to add this to turkey and cheese sandwiches or our burgers!

Kitchen Gear

Can opener

Strainer or colander

Sharp knife

Cutting board

Measuring spoons

Food processor

Rubber spatula or large spoon

Serving bowl

Ingredients

1 (16-ounce) can chickpeas (also called garbanzo beans), drained and rinsed with cold tap water

2 to 3 garlic cloves, peeled, and minced or chopped

3 tablespoons sesame tahini

1 tablespoon olive oil

3 tablespoons fresh lemon juice

½ teaspoon ground cumin, or more (if you like)

½ teaspoon kosher salt

¼ teaspoon black pepper

Lemon, lime, or orange slices, for garnish

Instructions

1. Put the chickpeas and garlic in the food processor fitted with a steel blade. Place the top on tightly and process until smooth.

2. Gradually, through the tube on top, add the tahini, oil, lemon juice, cumin, salt, and pepper and process again until completely smooth. If the hummus isn't completely creamy, add hot water 1 tablespoon at a time and process until it is.

3. Scoop the contents with spatula into the serving bowl, cover, and serve right away garnished with lemon slices, if using, and paprika. Can be refrigerated up to 3 days.

Classic Hummus *(cont)*

Personalize It

Try adding one of the following ingredients when you process the hummus:

- ½ cup chopped fresh basil, cilantro, or mint leaves

- ¼ cup chopped scallions, green and whites, or chives

- ½ cup chopped roasted bell pepper

- 1 tablespoon minced fresh chili peppers
  or ¼ teaspoon cayenne pepper

- ½ cup pitted green or black olives

- 1 tablespoon grated lemon, lime, or orange zest

Kids in the Kitchen

- Let your child add all of the ingredients to the food processor.

- Have her press the power button, and watch as the ingredients transform into a dip!

- Show your child how to garnish the hummus with lemon slices and paprika.

(Almost) Any Vegetable Soup

Hands-on time: 15 minutes
Total time: 2½ hours
Makes: 6 to 8 servings

This recipe works for almost any vegetable. You can also combine vegetables, if that's your fancy. If you like soup with a thick, creamy texture, add the rice or potato when you puree it.

Kitchen Gear

Measuring spoons

Sharp knife

Cutting board

Peeler

Can opener

Measuring cup

Large heavy-bottomed pot

Slotted spoon

Pot holder

Blender or food processor

Clean dish towel

Airtight storage container

Ingredients

1 tablespoon canola, vegetable, or olive oil or unsalted butter

1 large onion, coarsely chopped or thinly sliced

1 carrot, scrubbed or peeled, and chopped

1 celery stalk, sliced

1 garlic clove, peeled, and minced or chopped, or put through a garlic press

2 to 2½ pounds squash (butternut, winter, or summer) or button mushrooms, 1 bunch celery, or 2 (28-ounce) cans whole tomatoes or additional carrots

8 cups low-sodium chicken broth

¼ cup brown rice or 1 potato, scrubbed and cubed (if you like)

Instructions

1. Place the pot on the stove and turn the heat to medium. When it is hot, carefully add the oil.

2. Add the onion, carrot, celery, garlic (if using), and vegetables you have chosen and cook, stirring frequently, until the carrot is tender, about 10 minutes.

3. Add the chicken broth and rice or potato (if using), raise the heat to high, and bring to a boil.

4. Lower the heat to low and cook uncovered for 45 minutes. Set aside to cool down a bit, at least 15 minutes at room temperature or up to overnight in the fridge.

5. Very carefully, remove about 2 cups of the vegetables and 1 cup liquid from the soup and put them in the blender. Do not fill the blender more than halfway.

6. If using a blender, put the top on but remove the little cap in the center (this will allow the steam produced from the hot liquid to escape). Cover the cap hole with a clean dish towel. Turn the blender to the lowest speed and increase the speed as the soup purees. (If using a food processor, leave the plunger out while you puree the soup.)

(Almost) Any Vegetable Soup *(cont)*

Instructions *(cont)*

7. As soon as the soup is pureed, pour it into another pot or an airtight storage container. Repeat this same process until all the soup has been pureed. If you need to reheat the soup, pour it back into the pot and reheat over low.

8. Serve right away or cover and refrigerate up to 3 days.

Personalize It

Taste test and choose whatever vegetables you'd like to add to your soup.

Kids in the Kitchen

- Count their ingredients—do they have enough of each vegetable?
- Let your child add and mix all the ingredients into the pot.
- Have your child measure and pour the ingredients into the blender.

The Salad

Hands-on time: 20 minutes
Total time: 30 minutes
Makes: 4 burgers

If you can make salad dressing, you can make an amazing salad. Don't just think about iceberg and romaine lettuce: Be brave! Be daring! There are tons of salad greens to choose from. Below we list a lot of greens and try to explain what they taste like. And, below that, we offer a list of other fresh, delicious ingredients you might consider adding to your salad. The best salads include all kinds of flavors and textures, including salty, sweet, crunchy, and creamy. Simply open your mind before you open your mouth!

Personalize It

Greens

Arugula: also called "rocket," peppery and spicy

Belgian endive: bitter and crunchy; great paired with strong, creamy cheeses

Bibb lettuce: mild and sweet

Boston lettuce: buttery, very soft leaves

Chervil: a licorice-tasting herb

Chicory (curly endive): has a nice bite but can be slightly bitter to some

Cress: hot and peppery

Dandelion greens: nice and bitter (Warm the dressing to mellow it out.)

Endive: sweet, bitter, crunchy

Frisée: slightly sweet, slightly bitter; good paired with nuts and cheese

Green oak-leaf lettuce: mild and slightly grassy

Green chard: spinach-like (Use baby leaves for salad.)

Iceberg lettuce: crisp, mild, and delicious with blue cheese dressing

Mâche (also called lambs lettuce or corn salad): delicate flavor, best served alone

Mizuna: mustardy Japanese green

Mustard greens: crunchy, slightly bitter, and cabbage- like texture

Radicchio: beautiful deep red color; bitter and slightly peppery

Red chard (and beet greens): slightly sweet and grassy (Use baby leaves in salad.)

Red oak-leaf lettuce: mild and slightly nutty

Romaine lettuce: very crunchy, slightly sweet, slightly bitter

Watercress: peppery, spicy, great with citrus fruit

The Salad *(cont)*

Other Ingredients to Add to Salads

- Fresh fruit, including grapes, berries, sliced or diced apples, pears, peaches, nectarines, kiwi, mango, and sectioned tangerines, oranges, grapefruit, and clementines

- Dried fruit, including apricots, raisins, currants, cherries, figs, and dates

- Cooked and cooled (or leftover) vegetables, such as green beans, peas, asparagus, corn, cauliflower, and broccoli

- Fresh herbs, such as cilantro, basil, parsley, dill, chives, or mint

- Cooked, cooled, and sliced potatoes

- Tomatoes, any kind: cherry, beefsteak, plum, or yellow

- Raw vegetables, such as sliced or diced cucumbers, mushrooms, carrots, bell peppers, jicama, radishes, celery, and fennel

- Grated raw carrots or beets

- Pickled beets

- Roasted peppers

- Olives

- Sprouts, especially nice peppery ones such as broccoli or radish sprouts

- Thinly sliced onions, especially sweet ones like Bermuda, Walla Walla, or Vidalia

- Cheeses, almost any crumbled or grated, including feta, Parmesan, cheddar, blue, Brie, and goat

- Canned or marinated artichoke hearts

- Grilled or leftover chicken, beef, shrimp, or tofu

- Cooked beans, including black, white, chickpeas (also called garbanzo), red kidney, and pinto

- Toasted nuts or seeds

- Edible flowers, including borage, marigolds, violets, pansies, nasturtiums, and flowering herbs (Just be sure they're not sprayed.)

Salad Combinations

- Barley with sliced carrots, celery, and mushrooms

- Diced or sliced tomatoes, fresh herbs, and crumbled feta cheese

- Farro, chickpeas, diced tomatoes, crumbled feta cheese, and fresh mint

- Brown rice, shredded chicken, shredded cabbage, cilantro, and toasted sesame seeds

- Diced avocado and grapefruit

- Diced mango, avocado, and black beans

- Sliced or diced cucumber, peach, radish, and toasted walnuts

- Corn and black beans

- Diced celery, oranges, and feta cheese

- Strawberry, chopped asparagus, and avocado

- Cheddar cubes, diced apple, celery, and toasted walnuts

- Diced cucumber, radishes, and sesame seeds

- Grapes, toasted almonds, and shredded chicken

- Brown rice, shaved carrots, cucumbers, radishes, celery, onion, peas, and fresh herbs such as basil, mint, or parsley

Kids in the Kitchen

- Allow your child to taste test each ingredient before adding it to the salad.

- See how many ingredients you can add to the salad.

- Ask your child about the different textures and tastes of the salad.

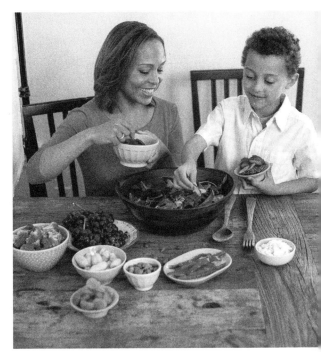

Rainbow Kabobs

Hands-on time: 5 minutes
Total time: 5 minutes
Makes: 1 kabob per person

"Eating the rainbow" helps get you in the habit of eating a full spectrum of fruits and vegetables—and, because different colors are associated with different nutrients, it's a great way to color your world healthy. What better way to get all your healthy hues than in a snack-able rainbow of fruit? Start with a container of fruit salad, if you like, or vary the ingredients to suit your taste.

Kitchen Gear	Ingredients
Sharp knife	Purple grapes
Cutting board	Blueberries
Bamboo skewers	Kiwis, peeled and cut into chunks
	Pineapple chunks
	Cantaloupe chunks
	Raspberries

Instructions

For each kabob, thread the fruit onto a skewer in rainbow order. Eat right away.

Personalize It

- Choose which fruits you'd like to add to your kabobs.
- Try other fruits such as mango chunks, strawberries, watermelon, and honeydew melon.

Kids in the Kitchen

- Taste test each ingredient before adding it to your kabob.
- Create a pattern with your fruits: sort them by color, shape, or taste!
- Count how many of each fruit you can add to your kabob.

Beanie Burger With Cheese

Hands-on time: 30 minutes
Total time: 30 minutes
Makes: 4 burgers

This is a great meal to serve vegetarians, of course, but it's also just plain great: tasty, satisfying, and full of nutrients. Serve the burgers with any of the following ingredients: lettuce, tomato, Guacamole (for recipe, see Chapter 6, page 184), salsa, Monterey Jack cheese, Cucumber Tsatziki (for recipe, see page 183), plain yogurt or sour cream, and lime quarters.

Kitchen Gear	Ingredients
Can opener	1 large egg
Colander or strainer	1 (16-ounce) can black beans, drained and rinsed with cold tap water
Measuring cup	½ cup leftover rice, barley, or panko bread crumbs
Sharp knife	2 scallions, greens and whites, minced (about ¼ cup)
Cutting board	2 tablespoons chopped fresh cilantro or basil leaves, or a combination
Measuring spoons	1 garlic clove, peeled, and minced or chopped (or put through a
Mixing bowl	garlic press)
Whisk	¼ teaspoon ground cumin
Fork	¼ teaspoon dried oregano or basil
Skillet	½ teaspoon kosher salt
Spatula	½ teaspoon black pepper
	1 teaspoon olive oil

Instructions

1. Crack the egg in the bowl and whisk until pale yellow. Add the beans and using the fork, mash until chunky.

2. Add the rice, scallions, cilantro, garlic, cumin, and oregano or basil to the egg and mix until well combined.

3. Divide the mixture into 4 portions and form each into a patty about ¾ to 1 inch thick. Sprinkle the patties with salt and pepper.

4. Place the skillet on the stove and turn the heat to high. When it is hot, add the olive oil. Add the burgers and cook until crusty on both sides and heated throughout, 4 to 5 minutes per side.

5. Top your burger with cheese and add a side of orange slices.

Beanie Burger With Cheese *(cont)*

Personalize It

Use other types of beans additionally or instead of black beans, such as

- Chickpeas (also called garbanzo)
- Pinto
- Dark red kidney beans

Kids in the Kitchen

- Show your child how to drain and rinse the beans using a colander or strainer.
- Let your child mash the bean mixture.
- Have your child form the beanie burger patties using his hands.
- Show your child how to flip the burgers using a spatula.

Oven-Roasted Broccoli

Hands-on time: 10 minutes
Total time: 20 minutes
Makes: 4 servings

Kitchen Gear

Measuring spoons

Vegetable peeler

Large-rimmed baking sheet

Sharp knife

Cutting board

Bowl

Pot holder

Heatproof spatula

Ingredients

1 large head broccoli

3 tablespoons olive oil

½ teaspoon salt

Lemon wedges, for serving

Instructions

1. Adjust an oven rack to the lowest position. Put the baking sheet on the rack. Turn the oven on and set the heat to 500 degrees Fahrenheit.

2. Peel the broccoli stalks as best you can. The thick peel will keep the broccoli from becoming fully tender, so you want to remove as much as you can.

3. Cut the stalk off the broccoli, and slice it into long, ½-inch, thick pieces. Cut the rest of the broccoli into long, fairly narrow florets (florets are the branched clusters at the top of the broccoli); then put it all in a bowl, drizzle it with the oil, and toss well until evenly coated. Sprinkle with the salt, and toss to combine.

4. Working quickly and carefully, use the pot holder to remove the baking sheet from the oven. Carefully transfer the broccoli to the baking sheet and use the spatula to spread it in an even layer.

5. Return the baking sheet to the oven and roast until the stalks are well browned and tender and the florets are lightly browned, 9 to 11 minutes. Serve right away with a little squeeze of lemon.

Personalize It

- Add chopped garlic.
- Add spices such as black pepper or red pepper flakes if you like it a little spicy.

Kids in the Kitchen

- Let your child peel the broccoli stalks.
- Have your child pull the florets off the broccoli from the stem.

Banana-Peach Frozen Yogurt

Hands-on time: 10 minutes
Total time: 10 minutes
Makes: 4 servings

According to the US Department of Agriculture, the most popular fruit in the United States is bananas, which can be found in most households. We recommend you keep a few sliced bananas (as well as berries) in your freezer so you can make this simple and speedy dessert anytime. If you don't have a food processor but have a blender, it's OK to use it. It's just a little harder to scoop everything out.

Kitchen Gear	**Ingredients**
Sharp knife	2 overripe bananas, thinly sliced and frozen
Cutting board	2 cups chopped frozen peaches
Measuring cup	½ teaspoon vanilla extract
Measuring spoons	⅓ cup plain yogurt
Food processor or blender	

Instructions

1. Put the frozen bananas and peaches in the bowl of the food processor fitted with a steel blade and put the top on tightly.

2. Turn the machine on and process until smooth. Gradually add the vanilla extract and yogurt and process until completely incorporated. Serve right away.

Personalize It

- Substitute mangoes or papaya for the peaches.

- Substitute fresh or frozen pineapple chunks and 1 teaspoon grated fresh lime zest for the peaches and vanilla extract.

- Substitute 4 cups frozen berries, including raspberries, strawberries, blueberries, and blackberries, for the peaches and bananas. Substitute 1 teaspoon lemon juice for the vanilla extract.

Kids in the Kitchen

- Taste test the ingredients before adding.

- Have your child add the ingredients to the food processor and turn on the power.

Double Corn Cakes With Fresh Corn

Hands-on time: 20 minutes
Total time: 35 minutes
Makes: 6 four-inch pancakes

Weekends, holidays, and summer can mean a little bit more time in the morning. If you aren't rushing off anywhere, try these delicious corn cakes for breakfast, topped with maple syrup and yogurt. Sound better for later in the day? They also make a great side dish for lunch or dinner, topped with summer salsa.

Kitchen Gear	Ingredients
Measuring spoons	6 tablespoons yellow cornmeal
¼ measuring cup	2 tablespoons whole-wheat or white flour
Large mixing bowl	¼ teaspoon baking soda
Whisk or fork	¼ teaspoon salt
Small bowl	¾ cup to 1 cup fresh or frozen corn kernels
Skillet	1 large egg
Spatula	¼ cup buttermilk or plain yogurt
	2 teaspoons canola oil

Instructions

1. Mix the cornmeal, flour, baking soda, and salt in the large bowl and combine with the whisk or fork. Set aside.

2. Combine the corn, egg, and buttermilk or ¼ cup yogurt in the small bowl and stir well.

3. Carefully pour the contents of the small bowl into the large bowl and mix well. Set the bowl aside for at least 15 minutes and up to 2 hours.

4. Place the skillet on the stove, turn the heat to medium, and let it heat up for 1 minute.

5. Very carefully add the oil.

6. Using the ¼ cup measuring cup, scoop the corn batter onto the hot skillet.

7. Use the spatula to gently push the blobs down to flatten them. This will make the pancakes thinner, which will help them cook faster and more evenly.

8. Cook the pancakes until the edges start to turn light brown and firm up. This will take about 2 minutes.

9. Once the edges are firm, flip the pancakes over and cook them for 1 more minute. When the pancakes are lightly browned on both sides, use your spatula to take them out of the pan.

10. Serve right away and add extra toppings for more flavor!

Double Corn Cakes With Fresh Corn *(cont)*

Personalize It

- Choose whatever topping you'd like for your corn cake, such as
  - Plain yogurt
  - Chives
  - Maple syrup
  - Summer salsa
  - Guacamole (For recipe, see Chapter 6, page 184.)

Kids in the Kitchen

- Allow your child to measure and add all ingredients to the mixing bowl.
- Have your child whisk the ingredients.
- Let your child scoop the mixture into the skillet and use the spatula to flip the corn cakes.
- Have your child pick out her toppings!

Vietnamese Chicken Noodle Soup

Hand-on time: 20 minutes
Total time: 45 minutes
Makes: 4 servings

Sour, spicy, crunchy, herbal, tender—this soup has just about every flavor and texture!
There are a lot of ingredients, but it's not hard to put together—and it's fun to serve and eat.

Kitchen Gear

Measuring cup

Sharp knife

Cutting board

Measuring spoons

Large pot

Wooden spoon or heatproof spatula

Pot holders

Large bowl

4 bowls, for serving

6 small bowls, for accompaniments

Ingredients

8 cups low-sodium chicken broth

4 quarter-sized slices fresh ginger

2 garlic cloves, peeled and thinly sliced

1 lemongrass stalk, thinly sliced

2 tablespoons fish sauce

4 ounces rice noodles

1 cup shredded or diced cooked chicken

¼ cup chopped fresh cilantro leaves

¼ cup chopped fresh basil leaves

1 cup bean sprouts

1 tablespoon Vietnamese chili paste (if you like it spicy)

1 lime, quartered

Instructions

1. Combine the broth, ginger, garlic, lemongrass, and fish sauce in the pot and place the pot on the stove. Turn the heat to high and bring to a boil. Once boiling, turn the heat down to low and cook 20 minutes.

2. While the broth is cooking, put the noodles in a bowl and cover them with hot water. Set aside until soft, 20 to 30 minutes. Drain the noodles and divide them among the 4 bowls.

3. Put the chicken, cilantro, basil leaves, bean sprouts, chili paste, and lime in individual bowls and place them on the table.

4. Ladle broth on top of each bowl of noodles and allow diners to add whatever they choose.

Vietnamese Chicken Noodle Soup *(cont)*

Personalize It

Allow your child to add whatever accompaniments he chooses!

Kids in the Kitchen

- Let your child measure and add each ingredient.

- Allow your child to mix the soup.

- Let your child squeeze the lime.

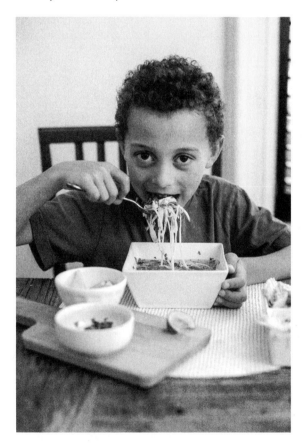

CHAPTER 4

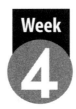

A Shopping Adventure

"You can't change the fruit
without changing the root."

— Stephen R. Covey,
author of *The 7 Habits of
Highly Effective People*

Mission
Change eating preferences by changing what is
available to eat.

Strategy
Stock the kitchen with healthy foods that are easy to make
that the family will actually eat.

Measurement
Parent and child perception of shopping experience.

"You can't change the fruit without changing the root." This observation came from the late Stephen R. Covey, author of the *7 Habits of Highly Effective People* and a leadership and parenting guru. He wasn't necessarily referring to changing kids' eating patterns, but he may as well have been. If parents really want to change the foods their kids eat, they need to change the home food environment. And that fundamentally begins with the grocery shopping and the food that is available in the home.

Although shopping with kids can sometimes (or always!) take longer and be a little more chaotic, the idea is that when kids are involved in making food choices, they tend to be more interested in trying those foods. For example, a child who gets to pick out one vegetable and one fruit for the family to eat during the week is more likely to help prepare that particular food and is more likely to eat it.

Shopping Trip Success: Brooke's and Hunter's Treasures

During their Picky Eater Project, Marlo and Corey decided to venture to a farmers market with their children. Farmers markets provide many rows of colorful displays, locally grown food that is in season and, thus, likely to be at its peak flavor. Kids are more likely to try foods when they are colorful and look delicious. If they realize they enjoy them, kids are more likely to add the item to their repertoire of acceptable foods. With school-aged kids, shopping at a farmers market offers another opportunity to apply additional learning to real life, such as math skills and budgeting.

On arrival, Marlo handed out $10 each to Brooke and Hunter and told them they could buy any vegetables and fruits they wanted. She suggested they shop around to get the best deal—after all, 2 vendors could both be selling strawberries each at a very different price. She also suggested they consider trying some samples if they came across anything that looked tasty or interesting. Eager shoppers, the kids bolted to a booth with gigantic pomegranates. Remembering these from a few weeks back when a neighbor had brought them over, she exclaimed that it's "one of the only fruits where you're supposed to eat the seeds!" Hunter bought 2 for $2, paid the vendor, counted his change, and put the fruit in his bag before he ran off to the next booth.

What happened next? Hunter came across a strangely shaped thing—a cucumber? He asked the farmer what in the world the thing was and where it came from. He learned that it was an Armenian cucumber, grown in the next town over, about 4 miles away. The farmer offered him a sample, which, to his parents' surprise, he eagerly obliged and gave it a try. He bought one for $1.

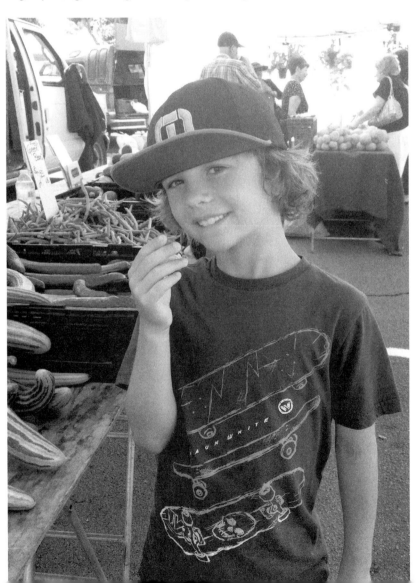

By the end of the shopping trip, Brooke had picked out green beans, guava, pears, and a kale plant (to feed to their pet bearded dragon). Hunter chose oranges, strawberries, persimmon, cucumber, the pomegranate and Armenian cucumber, and a zucchini, another vegetable he had never tried.

Once the kids got home, they snacked right away on the cucumbers and persimmons. Marlo and Brooke prepared to make an interesting new dinner—zucchini pasta with butter and Parmesan cheese, the kids' favorite type of pasta sauce. This recipe relied on a technique called bridging.

Bridging is a strategy used to help kids be willing to try new foods that are similar in taste or texture to foods they already enjoy. Hunter has already proven to like cucumbers. Zucchini is very similar to cucumbers. Both kids love pasta, so zucchini pasta seemed like the perfect recipe to try.

What happened next was a bit of a shock to everyone. The kids were not only willing to try the zucchini pasta but proved to love it just as much as regular pasta. In fact, when asked what part of this experiment had been the best so far, the whole family agreed that finding the zucchini pasta recipe was it.

A trip to your local farmers market promises to bring a colorful array of delicious, nutritious, inexpensive, and locally grown fruits and vegetables straight from the farm to your kitchen table, with little wasted time in between. Farmers markets are cropping up in communities across the United States. Make visiting a farmers market part of your Picky Eater Project, and see how your experience compares with Marlo and her family's.

Making the Most Out of Your Farmers Market Adventure

With these 10 tips, adapted from an article Natalie wrote for the American Council on Exercise, you're sure to not only have a great time but also set the stage for your kids to try a new food and broaden their preferences and hopefully add a new activity to your regular family routines.

❶ Find the best spot. Start your adventure online at www.localharvest.org, or a similar site. Here you can enter your zip code and obtain a listing of all the farmers markets in your area. In addition to times and locations, you also can get more information about each market, including what items are typically available (some even offer recipes, too).

❷ Make a list. While you are more likely to make spontaneous buys at a farmers market (because you never know exactly what you'll find there), it still helps to make a list of must-purchase items. Base this list off of your meal ideas for the rest of the week. This way you are sure to have a plan in mind of how you will prepare the great items you purchase at the market. Of course, once you arrive, be prepared to be flexible. Items move in and out with the seasons and you see what is or is not available. Another consideration is to shop first and then come up with your meal plan on the basis of an unexpected find.

❸ Invite your kids. Don't forget to grab your kids when you head out to the market! This is a wonderful opportunity to expose them to a wide array of healthy fruits and veggies that will look better and taste more delicious than what you normally pick up at the grocery store. With samples galore at many markets, this is a great time for them to try a bite of new foods they may otherwise reject.

❹ Bring reusable bags. In addition to connecting farmer to consumer, farmers markets also tend to advocate that we be good stewards of our environment. One easy way to do that is to remember to bring your reusable bags to cut down on plastic and paper bag waste.

5 **Walk or bike, if you can.** Keep up the spirit of optimizing your family's health by taking active routes to your local market, if possible. If you walk, consider taking a wagon or stroller to help transport your goods home. If you bike, make sure it includes a basket. If you must drive, make an extra effort to increase steps in your day by trekking through the entire market.

6 **Visit each booth.** Before you start buying, walk through the market to see what items are available and get a sense of costs. While you may think a farmers market is all fruits and veggies, this is not always the case. Many markets also include meat and fish, dairy products, processed foods, flowers, breads, and many other items. Visiting each booth is a great way to increase your physical activity, as well as get a feel for what is offered at what price. You will often find that 2 farmers may sell the same delicious fruit or vegetable for a notably different price.

7 **Sample, sample, sample.** One of the greatest perks of farmers markets is that you get a chance to sample a wide variety of items that you may not have ever considered buying. Sampling also gives you a chance to compare the taste of similar items from 2 different vendors. And—not to be forgotten—sampling offers your kids a chance to try new fruits and vegetables they may otherwise reject. It can take 15 to 20 times of tasting a previously rejected food for a child to actually come around to liking it. The experience of the market makes it more likely that your kids will be willing to give it a try. If they keep coming to the market, and they keep giving it a try, they may eventually come around to liking it!

8 **Learn about the farms.** Treat your outing to the farmers market as more than a chance to buy fresh food. Learn about the farms where the foods were grown as well. Encourage your kids to ask the farmers questions about what it is like to work on a farm or how to grow food. This will help transform your outing into a cultural experience.

9 **Go around closing time for the best deals.** Don't feel like you have to be the first one there. In fact, a little known secret is that many farmers will reduce prices (or be more open to bartering) near closing time. After all, most don't want to lug home the unsold food. Additionally, many farmers accept SNAP (Supplemental Nutrition Assistance Program) and WIC (Women, Infants, and Children) coupons or vouchers.

10 **Make a habit of it.** Make a visit to your local farmers market part of your family routines. You will benefit your community and local farmers, and the routine will go a long way toward optimizing your family's health and well-being.

Of Covey's 7 habits, the one most applicable to the grocery shopping experience and its role in undoing picky eating is number 2: "Begin with the end in mind." In other words, have a plan. This advice applies to many facets of everyday life, and the process of grocery shopping and its role in helping to raise healthier, more adventurous eaters is no exception.

This week you will stock your home with healthy foods that you not only *want* your kids to eat but also have a plan to present and prepare so they actually will. Just as you started this Picky Eater Project with an idea of what you hope to get out of it, we recommend that your approach to grocery shopping be the same. So let's get you started!

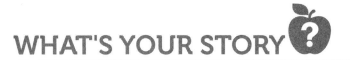

WHAT'S YOUR STORY

Your Own Farmers Market Adventure

Once you have checked out our 10 tips for shopping smart at the farmers market, start to plan for your own adventure. Divvy up some funds for each kid and let your kids choose what they'd like to get. Keep track of their picks and samples. Did anyone try anything new you'd never thought they'd go for? Were they more likely to eat an unfamiliar food they picked out at the market than one you just picked up at the store without their help?

Preschool Picky Eater Project

Christine and Fran, the parents of 4-year-old twins we introduced in Chapter 3 on page 68, had a similar positive experience with shopping with their twins, Nathaniel and Andrew. Fran, who works from home, routinely picks the boys up from preschool on Fridays. After preschool one day he decided he would take them to the grocery store and cook a twin-friendly dinner with their assistance. "We'll have turkey burgers," he said, "for the main course." They shouted in unison, "Yes!" He proposed that one pick a fruit and the other, a vegetable. Nathaniel shouted strawberries, while Andrew yelled apples and then potatoes. After looking through the vegetable section with his father, Andrew chose green beans instead.

Andrew and Nathaniel participated at every stage: shopping, forming the turkey into patties (after washing their hands), prepping the beans, measuring and pouring the oil, mixing ingredients, and spinning and ripping the lettuce. When they cooked the beans (see our Snappy Green Beans recipe on page 136), Nathaniel said, "I'm not going to have these because I don't love mustard." Andrew said, "I want it, I want it." When they sat down to dinner, Nathaniel objected to the toppings (onions, lettuce, and tomatoes), removed them, and then ate without commentary, as did Andrew. Additionally, Andrew tried the beans without being asked—but did not like them—which was still "a small victory" to Christine.

Grocery Store Shopping 101

❶ Start with a plan. Before heading to the store, we strongly suggest you have a plan of what you will need for meals and snacks for the family for the week. Then, write out a grocery list so you know what you need to buy. This will help save you time both in preparing meals and grocery shopping. Plus, you are more likely to have all the ingredients you need to quickly throw together a meal after a long day at work or taking care of the kids. To help get you started with this, check out our sample weekly meal plan and grocery list (Try It Out: Picky Eater Project Shopping 101).

Also, plan ahead for *when* you will go to the store. As much as possible, time it so shopping fits into your weekly routine and allows you to minimize time delays from traffic and other headaches, which could make the experience take longer and become more of a hassle.

❷ Involve the kids. While there is something to be said for a trip alone to the store to get everything done in time, as often as you can, take your kids along. Yes, it will slow you down a bit. Yes, you will have to brace yourself for the possible tantrum, the junk food item snuck into the bottom of the cart, and the momentary panic when you think you've lost a kid who snuck away while you were trying to corral her siblings. But the investment of time and energy you make now in helping your kids learn how to be smart and health-conscious shoppers will one day pay off at home. Table 4.1 includes developmentally tailored tips to make grocery shopping with the kids really fun.

TIP

A trip to the grocery store on an empty stomach or in a time crunch often ends with a hefty grocery bill and bags full of (unhealthy) foods that were not on the list. As much as you can, head out to the store when you have plenty of time and a relatively full stomach. Before you go, check for manufacturers' coupons and market specials and weekly promotions for items that are on your list. Also save money by comparing costs of similar items, buying fruits and vegetables in all their forms (fresh, frozen, canned, and dried), buying in bulk, doubling up recipes, and freezing extras for a later meal.

TRY IT OUT

Picky Eater Project Shopping 101

Use the Picky Eater Project Shopping Planner to help plan your weekly meals, snacks, and grocery list. Bring a copy to the store to make sure you don't miss anything (and also to help avoid impulse purchases).

Picky Eater Family Meal Adventures		
Dinner	**Other**	**Grocery List**
Mon	Breakfasts	
Tue		
Wed	Lunches	
Thu		
Fri		
Sat	Snacks	
Sun		

Table 4.1. Developmentally Tailored Tips to Make Grocery Shopping With the Kids More Fun
Involving the kids in grocery shopping is a really important piece of undoing the picky eating puzzle. With that said, we acknowledge that for many people shopping can feel like a chore. The thought of bringing your kids along may sound like an unwelcome suggestion. To help increase the likelihood of success, for kids of every age, make sure your kids are well rested and well-fed before the trip. A tired child will whine and a hungry child will fill your basket with unnecessary food. On the way there, set some ground rules, including what types of and how much foods they will be allowed to choose. Thank them in advance for following the ground rules, and offer to (nonfood) reward them for their good behavior. (Once the good behavior is the norm, the rewards are unnecessary and may even be a hindrance.) The following table lists a few ideas based on your child's age and developmental stage and may even help it to be fun and teach your child something while you're at it:

Age/Stage	Goal	Activity
Infancy	Expose your child to the sights, sounds, and words that will become a part of her everyday life as she learns to talk and experiment with her environment.	Boost your child's language development by pointing to and naming all the items you put into your grocery cart.
Toddler	A toddler's desire to exert control can be put to good use while also helping to get these resistant eaters to try new foods.	Give your toddler the power of choice by asking him to select a fruit and vegetable to make for dinner this week. Print out a picture of a few items you plan to buy at the store this week, laminate them, and challenge your toddler to try to find them at the store.
Preschool	Engage kids in the process of shopping to help increase awareness of different foods and the likelihood they'll want to try a wider variety.	Help your preschooler create her own preschool grocery checklist. Make a list of fruits and vegetables and other healthy foods your child would like to try or pick up at the store. Then put a drawing, sticker, or printed picture of each food next to the name of the food. Bring along this picture checklist to the store and encourage your child to find the foods and check them off of her grocery list. This not only keeps your child occupied but helps improve literacy and increase her knowledge of different types of foods.

Table 4.1 *(cont)*

Age/Stage	Goal	Activity
School	Teach kids about nutrition while also exposing them to various types of food.	Play games such as the MyPlate Grocery Store Treasure Hunt. Check out Figure 4.1 for a sample version. Play games such as grocery store bingo. Check out Figure 4.2 for our Picky Eater Project version.
Teen	Help your teen gain life skills, especially in learning how to select, purchase, and prepare ingredients to make balanced meals.	Ask your teen to choose one food from each of the following food types: • Fruit • Vegetable • Low-sugar dairy • Any type of seafood • A new "real food" they've never tried (ie, not processed) Challenge your teen to come up with a meal to make for the family one night per week. Create a grocery list together and head to the store to pick out all the needed ingredients. Ask your teen to devise a consistent MyPlate-inspired lunch plan for the week (Figure 4.3) and purchase all the items needed to follow through on it.

Figure 4.1. MyPlate Grocery Store Treasure Hunt

Reproduced from US Department of Agriculture Food and Nutrition Service. *Team Nutrition Popular Events Idea Booklet.* Washington, DC: US Department of Agriculture; 2014. Publication FNS-462. http://www.fns.usda.gov/sites/default/files/TNevents_appendixrepro6.pdf. Published March 2014. Updated January 13, 2016. Accessed March 7, 2016.

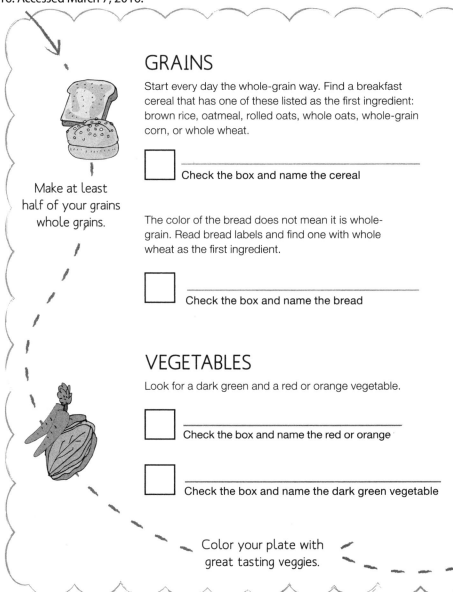

Make at least half of your grains whole grains.

GRAINS

Start every day the whole-grain way. Find a breakfast cereal that has one of these listed as the first ingredient: brown rice, oatmeal, rolled oats, whole oats, whole-grain corn, or whole wheat.

☐ Check the box and name the cereal

The color of the bread does not mean it is whole-grain. Read bread labels and find one with whole wheat as the first ingredient.

☐ Check the box and name the bread

VEGETABLES

Look for a dark green and a red or orange vegetable.

☐ Check the box and name the red or orange

☐ Check the box and name the dark green vegetable

Color your plate with great tasting veggies.

Families and Friends:

Take this sheet along with you the next time you go to the supermarket, and have your child look for foods in each food group. Make this a fun treasure hunt and a memorable activity for your child.

FRUITS

Find a fruit. If you choose a fruit juice, make sure it is 100% juice.

☐ _____
Check the box and name the fruit

Fuel up
with fruit.

DAIRY

Dairy foods contain calcium for strong bones and teeth. Find a dairy food that is low-fat or fat-free.

☐ _____
Check the box and name the dairy food

Get your
calcium-rich
foods.

MEAT AND BEANS

Try fish, shellfish, beans, and peas more often. Find a bag of dry beans.

☐ _____
Check the box and name the beans

Vary your
proteins.

Figure 4.2. Picky Eater Project Grocery Store Bingo

Carrots 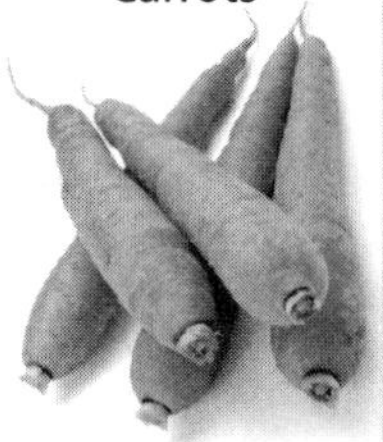	Eggs 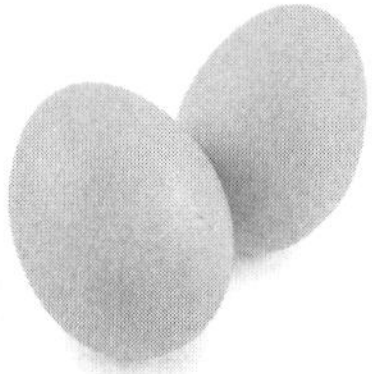	Frozen strawberries 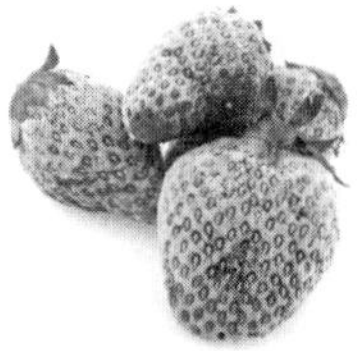	Walnuts 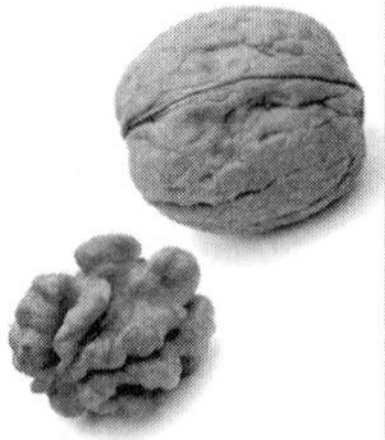	Whole-grain bread 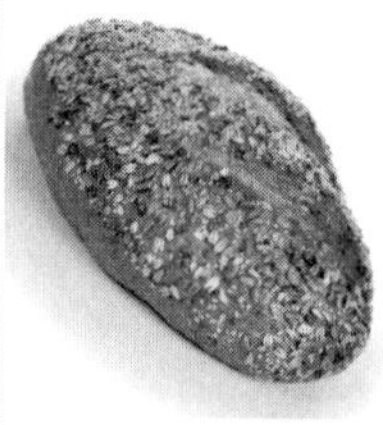
Blueberries 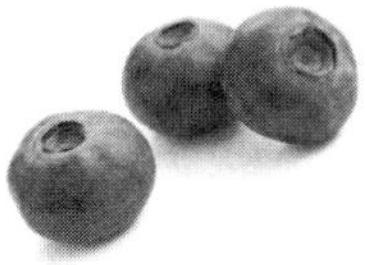	Basil 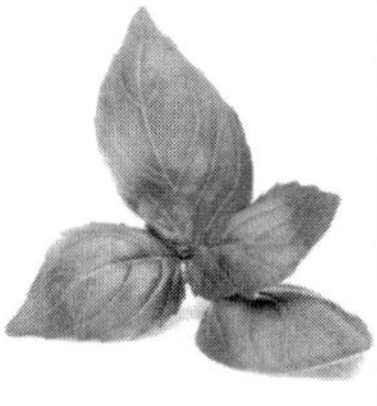	Apple 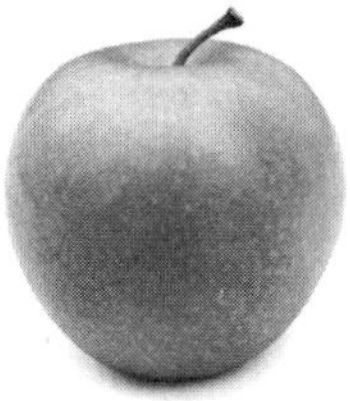	Cheddar cheese 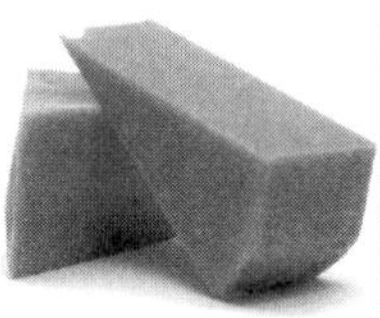	Grocery bag 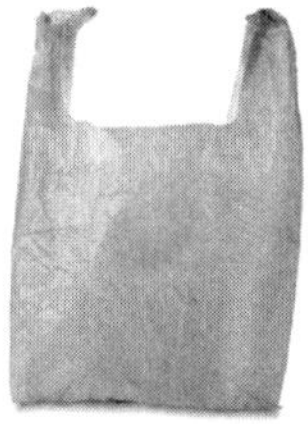
Cereal (with <5 grams of sugar)	Spinach 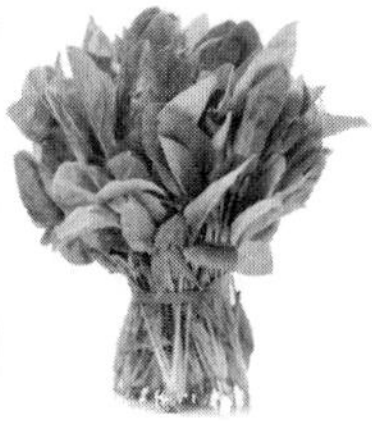	FREE	Artichoke 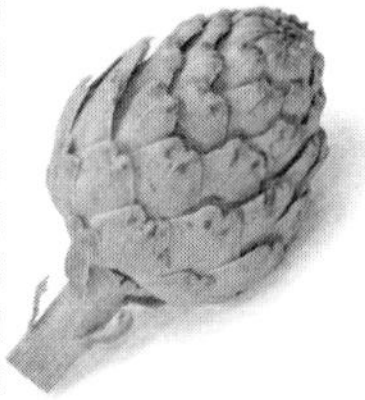	Zucchini 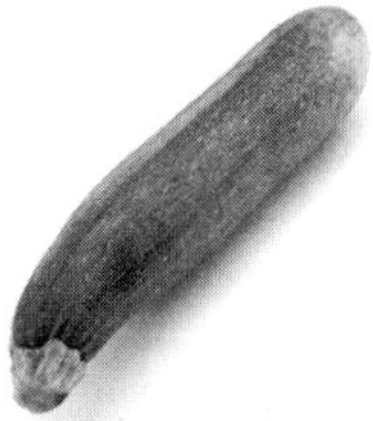
Fresh flowers 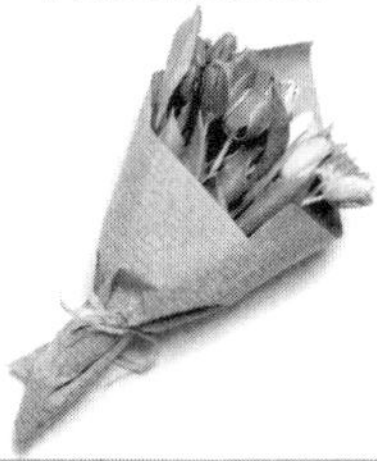	Store clerk 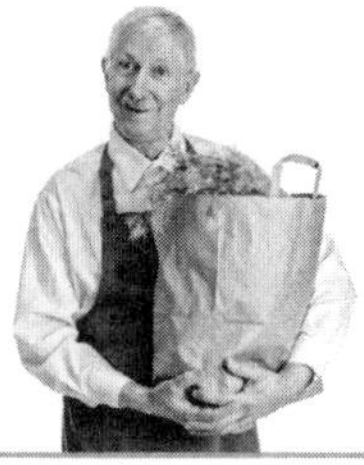	Salmon 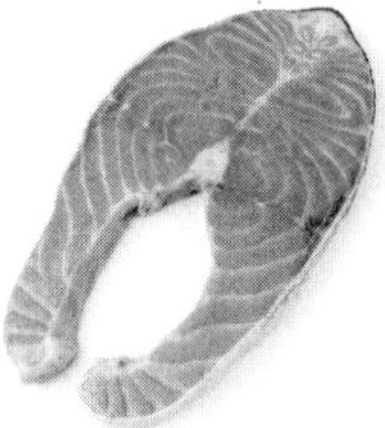	Canned tuna 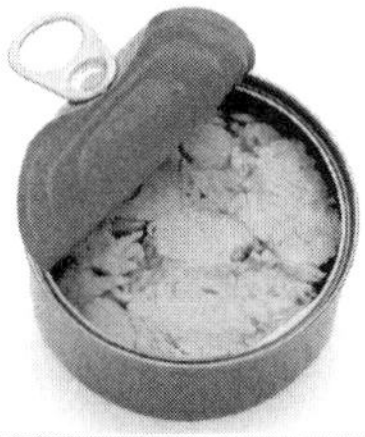	Diced tomatoes 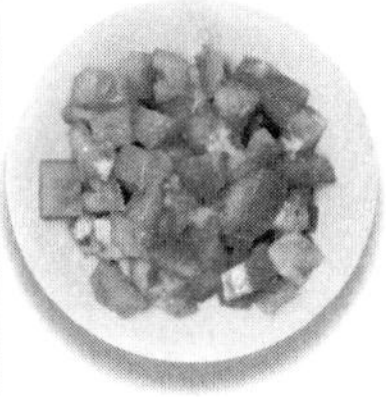
Almond milk 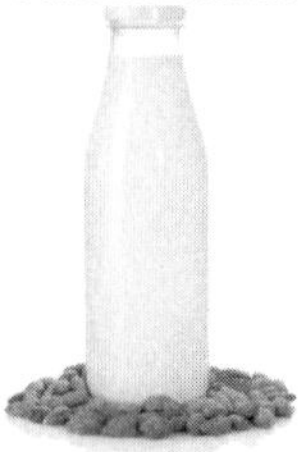	Banana 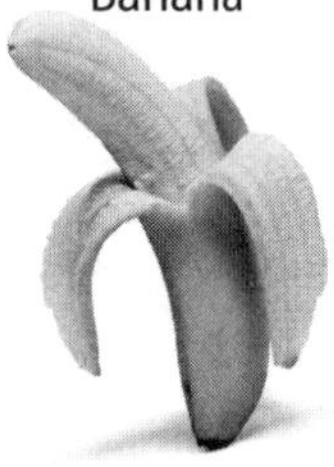	Olive oil 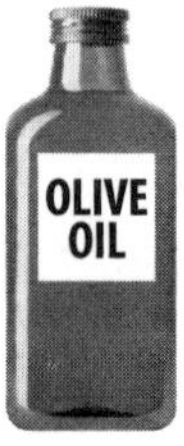	Couscous 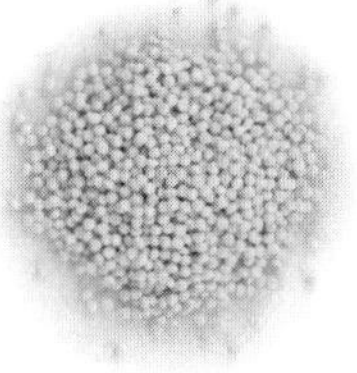	Cooking magazine 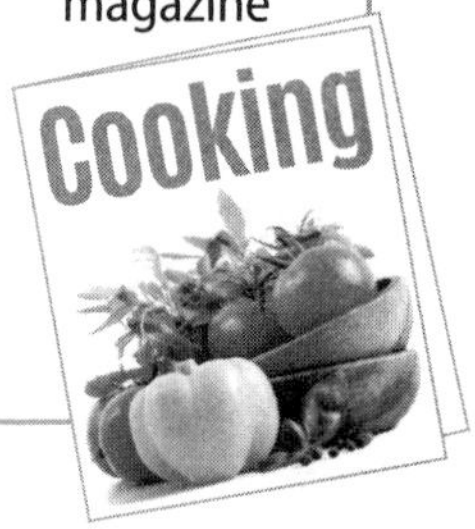

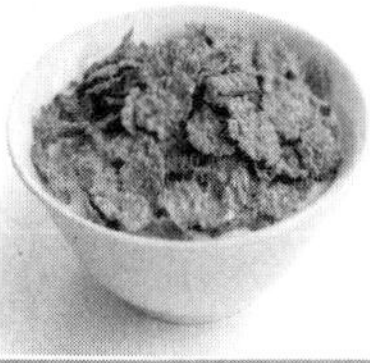

Figure 4.3. MyPlate

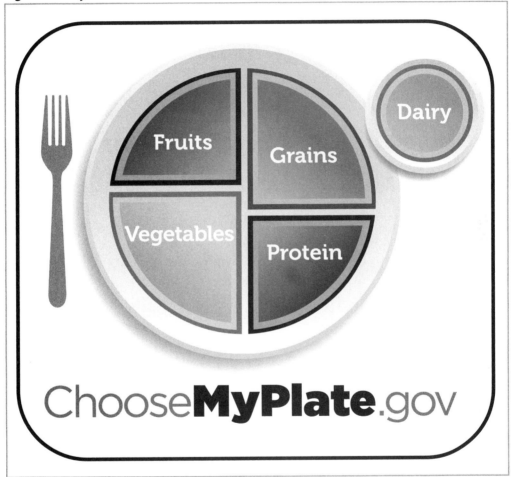

Reproduced from US Department of Agriculture. ChooseMyPlate Web site. http://www.choosemyplate.gov. Accessed July 25, 2016.

❸ **Review the Picky Eater Project Grocery Shopping Guide.** Grocery shopping offers a bombardment of choices. Even if you have a list, there are unlimited distractions, decisions to be made between 2 similar products to purchase, and constant strategic prompts and triggers to influence you to make an impulse buy. We've created the Picky Eater Project Grocery Shopping Guide in Table 4.2 to help you have a more successful experience.

Table 4.2. Picky Eater Project Shopping Guide

Food Group	Typical Store Locations	Best Choices
Vegetables and fruits	Produce aisle Canned goods Freezer aisle Salad bar	Variety! Fresh, frozen, canned, and dried fruits and vegetables. All forms have nearly identical nutrient value. Choose canned fruit in its own juice to minimize added sugars. Choose low-sodium and rinse canned vegetables first to further decrease sodium content. Watch portion sizes on dried fruit, as they are not only nutrient dense but also calorie dense. Whenever possible, it is best to choose locally grown, in-season produce. Check out our Picky Eater Project Produce Buying Guide in Table 4.3 for more information. When deciding whether to buy organic, we suggest using the Environmental Working Group guide. The "dirty dozen" (In other words, try to buy these organic, because of the relatively high pesticide exposure when grown conventionally.) • Celery • Peaches • Strawberries • Apples • Cherry tomatoes • Nectarines • Sweet bell peppers • Spinach • Tomatoes • Cherries • Cucumbers • Grapes (imported) The "clean 15" (lowest in pesticides; don't need to buy organic) • Onions • Avocado • Sweet corn (frozen) • Pineapples • Mango • Sweet peas (frozen) • Asparagus • Kiwi fruit • Cabbage • Eggplant • Cantaloupe (domestic) • Watermelon • Grapefruit • Sweet potatoes • Honeydew melon

Table 4.2 *(cont)*

Food Group	Typical Store Locations	Best Choices
Grains	Bakery Bread aisle Pasta and rice aisles Cereal aisle	Try whole-grain bread, brown rice, barley, bulgur, and quinoa. True whole grains will typically have the words *whole grain* as the first ingredient on the package's ingredient list.
Milk, yogurt, and cheese (calcium-rich foods)	Dairy case Refrigerated aisle	Need help deciding what milk to buy? Check out our milk guide in Table 4.4. Prefer nondairy sources of calcium? Try salmon, almonds, brazil nuts, sunflower seeds, dried beans, or calcium-fortified foods such as soy milk, tofu, and various breads.
Meat and beans, fish, poultry, eggs, soy, and nuts (protein foods)	Deli Meat and poultry case Seafood counter Egg case Canned goods Salad bar	The leanest forms of red meat are the round and loin cuts. Poultry such as chicken and turkey is an excellent protein source with low-fat content. Include fish in your family's meal plan for optimal health. Fatty fish provide high levels of omega-3 fatty acids, which help boost heart and brain health. These fish include salmon, albacore tuna, and lake trout. Wondering whether it's better to choose farmed or wild-caught fish? The answer of what's best varies. Look up the fish you are considering and get recommendations on what is healthiest and most environmentally conscious at **www.seafoodwatch.org.**

Table 4.3. Picking In-Season Produce

Taste is the most important predictor of whether a child likes a food. Increase the chances of a successful experience by choosing fruits and vegetables at their best—when they are most likely to taste delicious. The table below indicates the prime growing season for the most popular fruit and vegetables along with a description of how to pick the best one out of the bunch.

Fruit/Vegetable	January	February	March	April	May	June	July	August	September	October	November	December	The best fruit/vegetable is…
Apple													firm with no soft spots
Apricot													golden yellow, plump, and firm. Not yellow or green, very hard or soft, or wilted
Artichoke													plump and compact; green, fresh-looking scales
Asparagus													straight, tender, deep green stalks with tightly closed buds
Avocado													firm but yields to gentle pressure
Banana													firm with no bruises
Bell pepper													firm skin and no wrinkles
Blueberries													firm, plump, brightly colored
Broccoli													dark green bunches
Brussels sprouts													tight outer leaves; bright green color and firm body
Cantaloupe													slightly golden with light fragrant smell
Carrots													deep orange; not cracked or wilted
Cauliflower													bright green leaves enclosing firm and closely packed white curd
Celery													fresh, crisp branches with light green to green color

Table 4.3 *(cont)*

Fruit/Vegetable	January	February	March	April	May	June	July	August	September	October	November	December	The best fruit/vegetable is...
Cherries													firm, bright red
Coconut													heavy, free of cracks and mold, inside milk still fluid when coconut is shaken
Cranberries													firm, plump, brightly colored
Corn													green, tight, and fresh-looking husk; ears with tightly packed row of plump kernels
Cucumber													firm with rich green color and no soft spots
Eggplant													firm, heavy, smooth, uniformly dark purple
Grapefruit													firm, well rounded, heavy for size. Avoid puffy/rough skinned
Grapes													firm, plump, well-colored clusters
Honeydew													creamy yellow rounds and pleasant aroma
Kiwi													soft
Lettuce													fresh, crisp leaves without wilting
Mushrooms													firm, moisture and blemish free
Onion													dry and solid with no soft spots or sprouts

Table 4.3 *(cont)*

Fruit/	January	February	March	April	May	June	July	August	September	October	November	December	The best fruit/vegetable is...
Orange	▪	▪	▪	▪	▪						▪	▪	firm, heavy for size, and brightly colored skin
Peach					▪	▪	▪	▪	▪				soft to touch with fragrant smell
Pear	▪	▪			▪			▪	▪	▪	▪	▪	should yield gently to pressure at stem end
Peas			▪	▪	▪	▪	▪						bright green, full
Peppers						▪	▪	▪	▪	▪			firm with thick flesh and glossy skin
Persimmon	▪	▪							▪	▪	▪	▪	firm, plump, orange-red
Pineapple	▪	▪	▪	▪	▪	▪							slightly soft. Ripe when you can easily remove leaves with small tug
Plum					▪	▪	▪	▪	▪				plump, yield to slight pressure
Pomegranate									▪	▪	▪	▪	thin-skinned, bright purple-red
Spinach			▪	▪	▪	▪							large, bright leaves. Avoid coarse stems
Strawberries				▪	▪	▪	▪						dry, firm, bright red in color
Summer squash						▪	▪	▪	▪				firm with bright and glossy skin
Sweet potato	▪								▪	▪	▪	▪	firm, dark, smooth
Tomato						▪	▪	▪	▪	▪			plump with smooth skin and no blemishes

Reproduced with permission from Healthy Learning. Original source: Muth ND. *Eat Your Vegetables! and Other Mistakes Parents Make: Redefining How to Raise Healthy Eaters.* Monterrey, CA: Healthy Learning; 2012.

Table 4.4. The Picky Eater Project Milk Guide

The milk aisle used to have a couple of variations of cow's milk, but now there's an abundance of types of milk to choose from. Check out our milk guide below to choose which type is best for you and your family.

Milk	Nutrient Highlights (per 8 ounces)	Pros	Cons
Cow's milk (conventional) (skim, 1%, 2%, whole)	80–150 calories 0–5 grams saturated fat 8 grams protein 30% calcium 20% vitamin D	Skim milk is low in calories and fat and high in protein, calcium, and vitamin D. Choose skim or 1% low-fat milk for kids older than 2 years.	Lactose (problem for some) High carbon footprint, but industry working to lower
Organic cow's milk (skim, 1%, 2%, whole)	80–150 calories 0–5 grams saturated fat 8 grams protein 30% calcium 20% vitamin D	Same benefits as conventional milk	Expensive Lactose (problem for some)
Chocolate milk (1% low-fat)	150 calories 2 grams saturated fat 8 grams protein 29% calcium 18% vitamin D	More palatable than regular milk for some (especially appealing to kids)	11 grams added sugar per cup
Soy milk	100 calories ½ gram saturated fat 7 grams protein 29% calcium 16% vitamin D	Plant compounds may help decrease cholesterol.	Because soy contains estrogens, there was thought to be a theoretical risk it could increase breast cancer, but studies have not confirmed this to be true. The relationship between soy and health is an area of active research.
Almond milk	35 calories 0 grams saturated fat 1 gram protein 20% calcium 25% vitamin D	Lowest in calories High in vitamin E and selenium	Highest in sodium (180 milligrams per 8-ounce serving) Low in protein

Table 4.4 *(cont)*

Milk	Nutrient Highlights (per 8 ounces)	Pros	Cons
Hemp milk	100 calories ½ gram saturated fat 4 grams protein 10% calcium (30% if fortified) 25% vitamin D	High in omega-3 fatty acids (900 milligrams per serving)	Relatively low in protein and calcium (unless fortified)
Oat milk	130–150 calories 0 grams saturated fat 4 grams protein 0% calcium (30% if fortified) 0% vitamin D	High in calcium and vitamin D, folic acid, and fiber (2 grams per serving)	High in calories and sugar Little to no calcium unless fortified
Coconut milk	80 calories 5 grams saturated fat 1 gram protein 10% calcium 30% vitamin D	Lowest in sodium; fairly low calorie and fortified with vitamin B_{12} (especially important for vegans)	High in saturated fat Low in protein
Rice milk	120 calories 0 grams saturated fat 1 gram protein 1% calcium (30% if fortified) 25% vitamin D	Naturally sweet taste Low risk of allergic reaction	Low in protein

WHAT'S YOUR STORY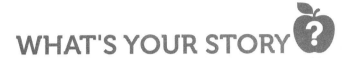

The Shopping Experience

Take your kids along on a shopping adventure, arming them with some of the tools and activities advised in this chapter, such as a preschool grocery checklist, a grocery store bingo, and the MyPlate Grocery Store Treasure Hunt. How did your shopping experience change? Did you notice they were more willing to pick out an unfamiliar food? Did they end up eating it once you got home?

Our shopping guide begins with MyPlate in mind (Figure 4.3). MyPlate recommends a balanced plate approach to healthy eating. That is, about half of what we eat should be vegetables and fruits; about a quarter, whole grains; and about a quarter, lean protein, plus dairy or a dairy substitute high in calcium and vitamin D, about 3 times per day. Sweets, candies, and desserts are best consumed sparingly (guidelines suggest that the typical child eat no more than 170 empty calories per day [calories with little to no nutritional value]).

We recommend most of your cart include vegetables and fruits, dairy and refrigerated items, and fresh meat and fish—items that you typically find in the outside aisles of the grocery store. If you minimize time you spend in the center aisles, you will purchase fewer of the highly processed foods that are usually shelved there. Of course, some healthy foods such as canned and dried beans canned tomatoes, and fish are shelved in center aisles, so we don't recommend avoiding them altogether. When you are shopping in center aisles or choosing packaged foods, be sure to read the nutrition label. Healthier options are lower in sugar and sodium and higher in fiber, vitamins, and minerals. Also, get in the habit of reading the ingredient list to make sure you are getting a quality food item.

Understanding the Nutrition Label

Learning how to read a nutrition label is an important skill for making smarter nutrition choices—although sometimes the best foods don't come with one! Processed foods are required by law to contain a package label describing the serving size, how many servings are in a package, and basic nutrition information related to calories, protein, fat, sugars, fiber, vitamins, minerals, and other nutrients. In addition, processed foods also contain an ingredient list. Together, this information is supposed to help a consumer make an informed decision, but historically it has been pretty challenging to make sense of the label. Recognizing this, in 2016 the US Food and Drug Administration approved a brand-new nutrition label, intended to make the process of choosing healthier foods easier. This new label will be on all packages by summer of 2018 and is described in detail in Figure 4.4.

How to Read the New Nutrition Label

❶ **Sizing up the serving information.** All the nutrient amounts listed on the food label are usually for one serving, so it is important to determine how many servings are actually being consumed to accurately assess nutrient intake. In the new nutrition label, the serving size listed is an amount of the food or beverage people tend to eat, not a recommendation of what they should be eating.

❷ **Total calories.** Calories are emphasized with a larger font, which makes it easier to compare similar food items.

❸ **Nutrient content.** Try to limit saturated fat, trans fat, and sodium. This part of the food label includes the total amount of sugars (natural and added) and now, with the updated label, added sugars. This is a critical and much needed addition for families looking to decrease sugar intake.

4 **Fiber and vitamins to calcium and iron.** Many kids don't eat enough dietary fiber, vitamin D, calcium, iron, and potassium. Kids generally need their age in years plus 5 grams of fiber per day. For example, a 2-year-old should eat about 7 grams of fiber per day. Eating a diet high in dietary fiber helps prevent constipation, a very common dietary issue in children, especially selective eaters. Additionally, a diet rich in fruits, vegetables, and grain products that contain dietary fiber, particularly soluble fiber, and are low in saturated fat and cholesterol if they replace fattier foods may reduce the risk of heart disease. Calcium and vitamin D are important for bone health, while potassium helps lower blood pressure. Iron is important for making hemoglobin to prevent anemia; if you're not anemic, it allows your brain to develop and allows you to be active. The old label included vitamins A and C, which food manufacturers may still list voluntarily. Vitamin A helps maintain healthy eyes, skin, bone, and teeth. Vitamin C is an antioxidant that helps promote healing, maintain healthy skin and bones, and absorb iron. Most kids eat enough vitamins A and C.

5 **Note the footnote.** The footnote at the bottom of the label reminds consumers that all % daily values (DVs) tell you how much of a nutrient a serving of food contributes to a daily diet, based on a 2,000 kilocalorie reference diet. While most teens need somewhere between 1,800 and 2,200 calories per day, younger kids need less. The typical 1-year-old needs about 900 calories; a 2- to 3-year-old, 1,000 calories; a 4- to 8-year-old, 1,200 calories; and a 9- to 13-year-old, 1,600 calories. While 3 grams of saturated fat provides 15% of the recommended amount for someone on a 2,000-calorie diet, it provides 30% for someone on a 1,500-calorie diet.

6 **The value of DVs.** The DVs are listed for key nutrients to make it easier to compare products, evaluate nutrient content claims (does one-third reduced sugar cereal really contain fewer carbohydrates than a similar cereal of a different brand?), and make informed dietary trade-offs (eg, balance consumption of a high-fat food for lunch with lower-fat foods throughout the rest of the day). In general, 5% DV or less is considered low, while 20% DV or more is considered high.

❼ Check for allergens. Food manufacturers must list all potential food allergens on the packaging. The most common food allergens are fish, shellfish, soybean, wheat, egg, milk, peanuts, and tree nuts. This information is usually included near the list of ingredients on the package. For those who follow a gluten-free diet, this is also an easy way to identify if wheat is a product ingredient.

❽ Ingredients list. Note that the ingredient list is in decreasing order of substance weight in the product. Thus, the ingredients listed first are the most abundant in the product. This list is useful for identifying the types of trans fat, solid fats, added sugars, whole grains, and refined grains that may be in the product. Note that although trans fat is included in the fats section of the nutrition label, if the product contains more than ½ gram per serving, the manufacturer does not need to claim it. However, if a product contains partially hydrogenated oils, then the product contains trans fat.

Solid fats: If the ingredient list contains beef fat, butter, chicken fat, coconut oil, cream, hydrogenated oils, palm kernel oils, pork fat (lard), shortening, or stick margarine, then the product contains solid fats. The Dietary Guidelines from the US Department of Agriculture advise limiting solid fats.

Added sugars: Ingredients signifying added sugars include anhydrous dextrose, brown sugar, confectioners' powdered sugar, corn syrup, corn syrup solids, dextrin, fructose, high-fructose corn syrup, honey, invert sugar, lactose, malt syrup, maltose, maple syrup, molasses, nectar, pancake syrup, raw sugar, sucrose, sugar, white granulated sugar, cane juice, evaporated corn sweetener, fruit juice concentrate, crystal dextrose, glucose, liquid fructose, sugar cane juice, and fruit nectar. In many cases, products contain multiple forms of sugar. Added sugars (which contain 4 calories per gram) should be limited to less than 10% of calories per day.

Whole grains: Whole grains have a particular whole grain listed as the first or second ingredient. Examples of whole grains include brown rice, buckwheat, bulgur (cracked wheat), millet, oatmeal, popcorn, quinoa, rolled oats, whole-grain sorghum, whole-grain triticale, whole-grain barley, whole-grain corn, whole oats/oatmeal, whole rye, whole wheat, and wild rice.

Refined grains: Refined grains are enriched. This means the grain has been heavily processed, removing the healthy nutrient-rich portion, and then some B vitamins are added back to the grain after processing. If the first ingredient is an enriched grain, then the product is not a whole grain. This is one way to understand whether a wheat bread is actually whole wheat or a refined product.

Food Label Tips

A lot of information is contained on the food label, and what to focus on depends mainly on the particular food and your goals. For example, when consuming snack foods, it is important to note the serving size and number of servings per container. The calories in a serving also are important to know to avoid overeating, as are sodium and sugar, which are ingredients to limit. If your child has a food allergy, reading the ingredient list is essential. When choosing grains, comparing fiber content is of value. Additionally, while the food label is found on the side or back of products, other health and nutrition claims are often visibly displayed on the front of the package. Though the US Food an d Drug Administration regulates these claims, they are fre-

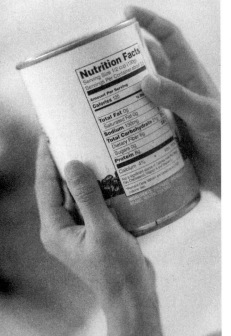

quently a source of confusion. Consumers should be skeptical of front-of-package claims and evaluate them on a case-by-case basis. A loophole allowing *qualified health claims* has paved the way for manufacturers to claim unproven benefits to products, as long as the label states the claim is supported by very little scientific evidence. As a general rule, if a food seems to be boasting how healthy it is on the front of the package, it probably isn't very healthy.

Also, beware of marketing traps. Chips and candy are placed in check-out lines to encourage an impulse buy. They create beautiful displays of less healthy food items so you will buy them. Go in aware of this and you will be less likely to fall in the trap.

Figure 4.4. The Nutrition Label

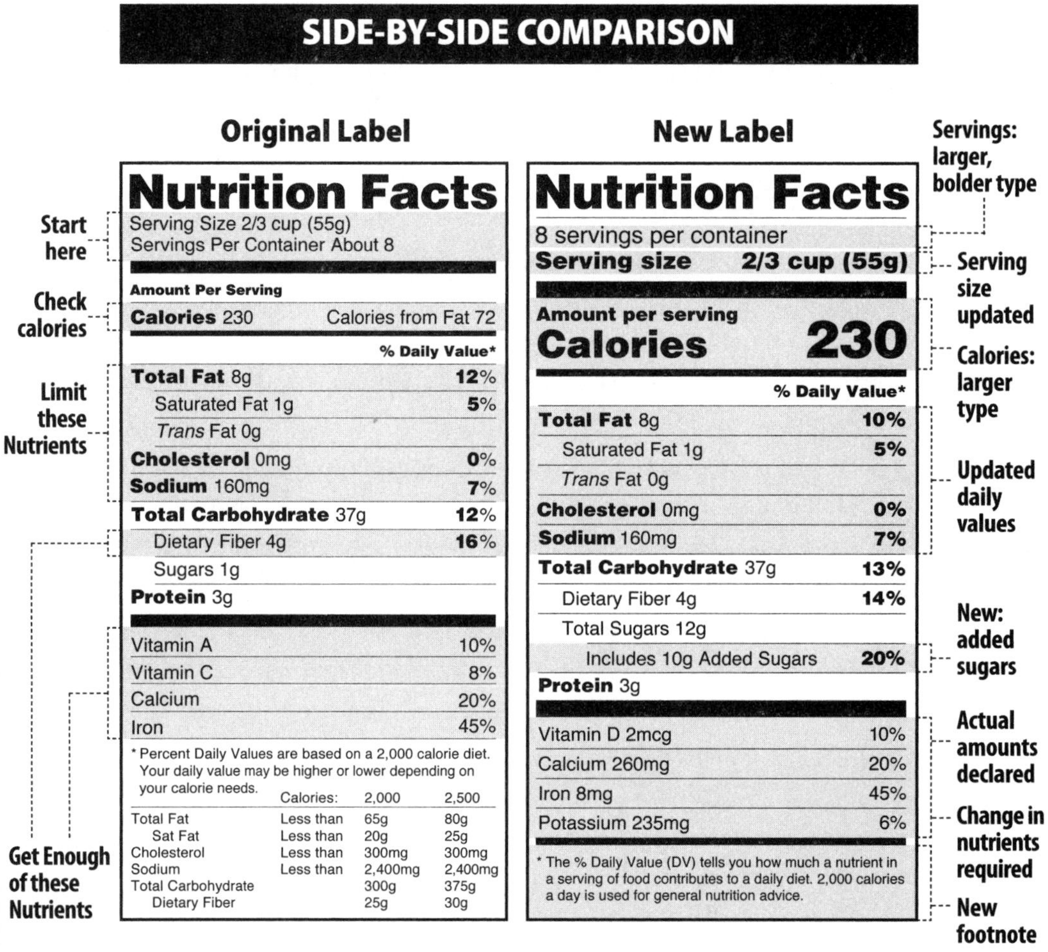

SIDE-BY-SIDE COMPARISON

Original Label

Nutrition Facts
Serving Size 2/3 cup (55g)
Servings Per Container About 8

Amount Per Serving

Calories 230   Calories from Fat 72

% Daily Value*

Total Fat 8g	12%
Saturated Fat 1g	5%
Trans Fat 0g	
Cholesterol 0mg	0%
Sodium 160mg	7%
Total Carbohydrate 37g	12%
Dietary Fiber 4g	16%
Sugars 1g	
Protein 3g	

Vitamin A	10%
Vitamin C	8%
Calcium	20%
Iron	45%

* Percent Daily Values are based on a 2,000 calorie diet. Your daily value may be higher or lower depending on your calorie needs.

	Calories:	2,000	2,500
Total Fat	Less than	65g	80g
Sat Fat	Less than	20g	25g
Cholesterol	Less than	300mg	300mg
Sodium	Less than	2,400mg	2,400mg
Total Carbohydrate		300g	375g
Dietary Fiber		25g	30g

New Label

Nutrition Facts
8 servings per container
Serving size   2/3 cup (55g)

Amount per serving
Calories   230

% Daily Value*

Total Fat 8g	10%
Saturated Fat 1g	5%
Trans Fat 0g	
Cholesterol 0mg	0%
Sodium 160mg	7%
Total Carbohydrate 37g	13%
Dietary Fiber 4g	14%
Total Sugars 12g	
Includes 10g Added Sugars	20%
Protein 3g	

Vitamin D 2mcg	10%
Calcium 260mg	20%
Iron 8mg	45%
Potassium 235mg	6%

* The % Daily Value (DV) tells you how much a nutrient in a serving of food contributes to a daily diet. 2,000 calories a day is used for general nutrition advice.

Labels (left side): Start here · Check calories · Limit these Nutrients · Get Enough of these Nutrients

Labels (right side): Servings: larger, bolder type · Serving size updated · Calories: larger type · Updated daily values · New: added sugars · Actual amounts declared · Change in nutrients required · New footnote

Note: The images above are meant for illustrative purposes to show how the new Nutrition Facts label might look compared to the old label. Both labels represent fictional products. When the original hypothetical label was developed in 2014 (the image on the left-hand side), added sugars was not yet proposed so the "original" label shows 1g of sugar as an example. The image created for the "new" label (shown on the right-hand side) lists 12g total sugar and 10g added sugar to give an example of how added sugars would be broken out with a % Daily Value.

Adapted from US Food and Drug Administration Web site. http://www.fda.gov/food/guidanceregulation/guidancedocumentsregulatoryinformation/labelingnutrition/ucm385663.htm. Accessed August 10, 2016

Change it up a little. While you may get most of your food from the local grocery store, you might consider trying some alternatives when it comes to choosing your produce. For example, visiting a farmers market, joining a community-supported agriculture (CSA for short) cooperative, or shopping from a local farm stand offers an opportunity to try fresh, homegrown produce. You are not only supporting local businesses and farmers but raising kids who are more likely to be willing to taste and like the food when it is fresh and locally grown—all factors that make it more likely the food is eaten at its peak ripeness and flavor.

Finally, once you have ventured out to the store, double-check your plan. How well did you stick to your list? Were your kids a help? In what one way did you help change the path ever so slightly to move in the direction of positive change at your home?

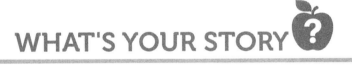

WHAT'S YOUR STORY

Practice reading nutrition labels next time you go to the grocery store. Here's a sample activity to help you.

The Cereal Aisle
Read labels and try to find 3 cereals that have < 5 grams of sugar per serving.

Yogurt
Search for a healthy yogurt for the children that is free of added sugars (review all the ways to say sugar in Table 2.2 on page 38).

The Snack Aisle
Visit the snack aisle and try to find a product that meets the healthy snack recommendations outlined in Table 2.3 on page 38.

YOUR PICKY EATER PROJECT—WEEK 4

A Shopping Adventure

Project To-dos Checklist

☐ Take the kids with to the store armed with their very own shopping list (see Table 4.2 on page 118, Picky Eater Project Shopping Guide, for grocery list ideas.). Help them navigate the store to find their items and cross them off the list. For older kids, incorporate math and budgeting skills by providing them a fixed amount of money to spend to get all the items on their list.

☐ Play grocery store bingo. Offer a nonfood prize like stickers or a new book when the kids get a bingo! (See Figure 4.2 on page 116.)

☐ Shop in a new place, such as a farmers market, through a community-supported agriculture cooperative, at a farm stand, or at other locale where you can purchase fresh, locally grown food.

Project Check-in

❶ You are halfway done with the Picky Eater Project! Check in on your progress. On a scale of 1 to 10 (1 being not very well; 10 being very well), how well do you think it's going? What will it take to move up on the scale next week?

❷ How was practicing your "picky-free parenting" rules this week, especially when faced with what can be a stressful experience (shopping with your kids)?

What was the greatest challenge in shopping with your kids? What was the greatest reward?

❸ On a scale of 1 to 10 (1 being the least enjoyable; 10 being the most), how successful was your shopping experience? Ask your children to rate the same. Discuss together what worked really well and what you might do differently next time to make it even better.

Week 4 Recipes

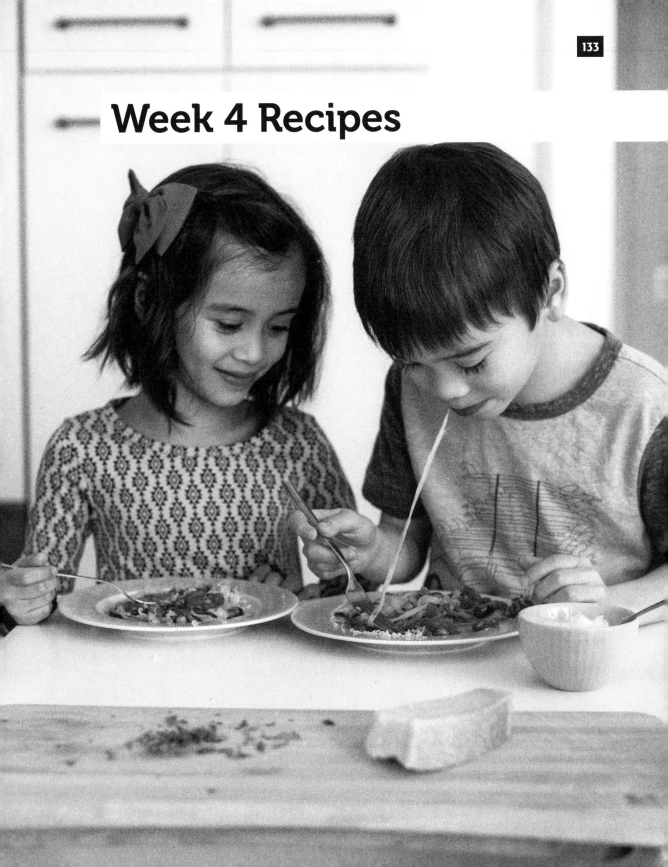

Zucchini Pasta

Hands-on time: 10 minutes
Total time: 15 minutes
Makes: 4 servings

Kitchen Gear

Measuring spoons

Sharp knife
  or spiralizer

Cutting board

Medium skillet

Ingredients

2 teaspoons olive oil

2 tablespoons water

2 zucchini, cut in very thin strips

Pinch salt

Finely grated Parmesan cheese

Instructions

1. Place a medium skillet over high heat. When it is hot, carefully add the olive oil and water.

2. Add the zucchini and cook, stirring occasionally, until the zucchini is tender and golden, about 5 minutes.

3. Serve right away, sprinkled with salt and Parmesan cheese.

Personalize It

- Make your own tomato sauce.

- Make your own pesto.

Kids in the Kitchen

- Carefully allow your child to cut the zucchini into thin strips using the spiralizer. Or, use a peeler!

- Let your child mix the zucchini while it's cooking in the skillet.

- Have your child choose and taste different cheese toppings.

Snappy Green Beans

Hands-on time: 20 minutes
Total time: 20 minutes
Makes: 4 servings

Green beans are also known as snap beans because of the snap sound they make when they are broken. Green beans can be used as a side dish or quick snack—and you can even eat them raw!

Kitchen Gear	Ingredients
Measuring spoons	1 pound green beans, ends trimmed
Colander or strainer	2 tablespoons olive or canola oil
Measuring cup	1 tablespoon Dijon or yellow mustard
Saucepan with lid	1 tablespoon red wine vinegar or fresh lemon juice
Mixing bowl	
Fork or spoon	

Instructions

1. Place the colander or strainer in the sink.
2. Place 2 cups water into the saucepan, cover, and bring to a boil over high heat. Turn the heat off.
3. Add the beans to the saucepan and let them sit in the water until they turn bright green, about 10 minutes.
4. Pour the beans into the colander or strainer and then let cold water run over them until completely cooled.
5. Place the cooled beans into the mixing bowl; add the oil, mustard, and red wine vinegar or lemon juice; and mix together with the fork or spoon.
6. Serve the beans right away or cover and refrigerate overnight.

Personalize It

- Add fresh chopped herbs like basil or cilantro at the end.
- Add lime juice instead of lemon juice.

Kids in the Kitchen

- Let you child measure and add each ingredient.
- Allow your child to trim off the ends of the beans.
- Let your child squeeze the lime.

CHAPTER 5

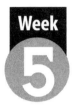

Family Mini-feast

"If we want our kids
to lead healthier lives, we need
to eat with them more often."

— Miriam Weinstein, author of
*The Surprising Power
of the Family Meal*

Mission
Eat more pleasant meals together.

Strategy
Model healthy habits through family mealtimes.

Measurement
Number of meals eaten together as a family.

While prior to the Picky Eater Project family meals may have consisted of 3 or 4 separate meals depending on each family member's mood and preferences, Marlo and Corey have always made family meals a priority at their house. While everyone may not always eat the same thing, they all sit down together most nights. The TV is off; no phones, tablets, or other devices are allowed. About 4 nights out of the week, the family eats together at the dining room table; 2 nights, at the kitchen table; and the other night, usually out or when Marlo has to work, so the rules are a little relaxed (ie, TV might be in the background).

In fact, it is because the family ate so many meals together that it became apparent to Marlo and Corey that something had to change with how they went about choosing and preparing food for these family meals. It's not sustainable to throw together 2 or more full dinners each night, just to keep everyone happy and well-fed. We didn't need to convince the family this week why family meals are so important, but we did get a chance to emphasize some of the benefits that can come when everyone is not only together but also eating the same foods.

Marlo and Corey agreed intellectually with this idea, but they still struggled when one or both kids would refuse or be uninterested in eating what was offered.

"It's kind of a free-for-all after dinner if we didn't like or want what was made," Brooke commented.

Despite our reassurances that their kids would come around, Marlo and Corey continued to share the strong belief that their kids should not go to bed hungry if they have refused dinner.

The good news is that the benefits that come from eating meals together as a family still add up, even if everyone is not necessarily eating the same thing. Family meals offer an excellent opportunity for parents to model not only what to eat but also how to eat—including balanced meals, controlled portions, being open to new tastes and textures, learning manners and social norms around eating, and being connected and engaged with one another. The science is clear: frequent family meals equals healthier eaters, especially when the parents are generally healthy and adventurous eaters themselves. Kids who eat at least 3 meals per week with at least one adult family member eat fewer sweets, fried foods, and soda and more vegetables, fruits, and other nutritious foods. In case you need further convincing, those who regularly eat meals with their families not only are healthier and less likely to be affected by childhood obesity but also perform better in school, develop advanced language skills, and are less likely to drink alcohol or experiment with other drugs as teens.

The benefits of family meals are most pronounced if everyone eats the same meal—and if the meals offered are balanced and readily accepted by all family members. But big changes don't happen overnight. This week we reinforced the positive family mealtime rituals that Marlo and Corey practiced and worked with them to restructure dinners to make it more likely the whole family would be able to come together and eat the same meal.

For Marlo and Corey, the biggest challenge is just that: getting everyone to eat the same meal. But we acknowledge that there are many additional potential obstacles can get in the way of eating a meal together as a family—for example, too many schedules to coordinate, pressures on time, picky eating preferences, pure exhaustion from the daily grind. Our goal is to help you chip away at these barriers and make it easier to eat the same dinner together as a family most nights. As you do this, you will find that your child's picky eating preferences become less pronounced and eventually (be patient!) not apparent at all. We will do this through a 5-step plan that we challenge you to try to implement this week.

The Picky Eater 5-Step Plan

❶ Step 1. Make the commitment. This sounds obvious and simple enough, but if you don't commit to *at least 3 meals per week* together (or whatever number is doable at your house), barriers to eating together will become overwhelming and you may fall into old habits. Choose a goal number of family meals to eat together this week, and do everything in your power to achieve that goal.

② **Step 2. Set a time for dinner.** Choose a time when everyone is most likely to be present, even if that means you push off dinner until 7:30 pm or eat earlier at 4:00 pm or 5:00 pm. Kids can adjust snack times and amounts to make sure they're hungry (but not "starving") for dinner. If at all possible, plan your work schedules so at least one parent is home for a sit-down dinner on most nights. Think twice before signing your child up for an activity that will extend into dinnertime. At all costs, try to avoid having your child eat dinner alone.

③ **Step 3. Plan ahead.** For many people, the chances of coming home after a long day of work and exerting the mental focus and energy to think up what to make for dinner and then find all the right ingredients are slim to none. Avoid this problem by spending an hour once a week to brainstorm a menu of meals for the coming week. Consider putting together a family calendar where you write down every-

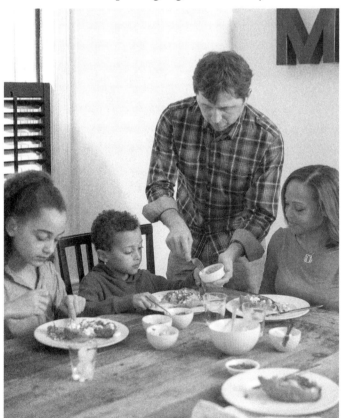

one's activities as well as the planned menu for each day (review Try It Out: Picky Eater Project Shopping 101 in Chapter 4 on page 110 for a weekly meal planning template). This way everyone knows what to expect and you can maximize the chances you'll be able to quickly put together a healthy meal (Box 5.1) for the family.

Box 5.1. Building Blocks of a Healthy Meal

As you plan healthy meals for your family, keep the following considerations in mind:

Half and half. Make half the plate vegetables and fruits. Vegetables and fruits are full of nutrients and help promote good health, especially red, orange, and dark green vegetables such as tomatoes, sweet potatoes, and broccoli. Even if your kids don't eat them, including fruits and vegetables at every meal and with snacks helps them become more familiar with these foods (and hopefully more likely to try them) and emphasizes what a healthy, balanced meal looks like.

Putting the "pro" in protein. Add lean protein. Include protein foods such as seafood, chicken, turkey, beans, tofu, lean beef, pork, eggs, or nuts at most meals. While most beans are not a "complete protein" (they do not contain all of the essential amino acids), that is OK. Generally, over the course of the day, the "missing" amino acids will be consumed through intake of other complementary foods, which include rice; other grains such as corn, wheat, and barley; and nuts and seeds.

Looking at the "whole" picture. Include whole grains as much as possible. Aim to make at least half of your grains whole grains. Look for the words 100% whole grain or 100% whole wheat on the food label. Whole grains provide more nutrients, such as fiber, than refined grains. If your kids are stuck on white grains, gradually transition them to whole grains first by choosing white whole-grain products or mixing half white and half whole grain (eg with pasta or rice). After they have accepted the initial shift, trial just the whole grain version.

Don't forget the dairy. Include a calcium-rich food. Pair your meal with a cup of milk, yogurt, or cheese to help offer enough calcium in your and your child's diet. Don't eat dairy? Salmon, almonds, brazil nuts, sunflower seeds, dried beans, and calcium-fortified foods such as soy milk, tofu, and some breads are also good sources of calcium.

Take it easy on the extras. Avoid extra solid fats. Using heavy gravies or sauces will add saturated fat and calories to otherwise healthy choices. Instead, aim to grill foods or use healthier fats such as olive oil when cooking.

Go slow. Encourage your kids to slow down and enjoy the taste and textures of their food, as well as pay attention to feelings of hunger and fullness. Encourage your kids to set down their forks with each bite and chew their food 10 or 20 times before swallowing. Eating quickly is associated with eating too much. Remember, it can take 20 minutes to feel full.

Box 5.1 (cont)

Less is more. Using a smaller plate helps with managing portion sizes and avoiding overeating. When we use larger plates, serving sizes increase and, consequently, actual food intake goes up.

Home sweet home. Take control of your food. Eat at home more often so you know exactly what you and your family are eating. Choose to cook healthier options such as baked items instead of fried.

Out of the comfort zone. Try new foods. Keep it interesting by picking out foods you've never tried before, like mango, lentils, or kale. You may even find a new favorite. Trade fun and tasty recipes with friends.

Be smart about sweets. Satisfy your sweet tooth in a healthy way. Indulge in a naturally sweet dessert dish—fruit! Serve a fresh fruit cocktail or a fruit parfait made with yogurt. For a hot dessert, try our Melting Apples recipe on page 153.

Need help figuring out how to put all of this together to create a meal plan for the whole day? See how it might work with our following 1-day meal plan example.

Breakfast. Scrambled eggs with cheddar cheese and tomatoes on a whole-wheat English muffin with a side of orange slices.

Snack. Apple slices.

Lunch. Nut or sunflower butter and banana sandwich on whole wheat paired with plain yogurt and strawberries. Or, try a school lunch mix and match to make prepping lunch even more fun (check out the Try it Out: School Lunch Meal Mix and Match on page 144).

Snack. Carrots and hummus. (For recipe, see page 85.)

Dinner. Fajitas, Fish Tacos, or Sweet Potato Bar (see pages 155, 157, and 159, respectively) or any of the other delectable recipes.

TRY IT OUT

School Lunch Meal Mix and Match

Engage your children in learning how to plan balanced meals with our school lunch mix and match activity. Place a mix of ingredients on the kitchen counter that includes whole grains, proteins, vegetables, fruits, and dairy or other calcium-rich foods. Prompt your kids to make a balanced school lunch from the ingredients provided (of course, your level of supervision will vary on the basis of your child's age). Ask them how they decided what balanced looks like:

Ideas for ingredients include

Grains	Proteins	Vegetable	Fruit	Dairy/ Alternatives
Whole-wheat bread, English muffin, bagel, or bun	Lunch meat (nitrite-free preferable)	Carrot sticks or baby carrots	Apple	Yogurt
Cooked pasta	Hard-boiled egg or egg salad	Edamame	Orange	Cheese stick
Cooked brown rice	Peanut butter/ almond butter/ sunflower butter	Snap peas	Banana	Cow's milk
Tortilla wrap	Hummus	Celery sticks	Pears	Almond milk
	Canned tuna or tuna salad	Sliced tomato	Dried fruit like raisins, cranberries, or apricots	Tofu
Pita	Grilled chicken	Avocado	Grapes	Cottage cheese
Whole-grain crackers	Mixed nuts	Sliced cucumbers	Berries	

Here are sample lunches your kids might come up with using these ingredients.

- Turkey sandwich on whole-wheat bread, orange slices, edamame, and a cheese stick
- Cooked whole-grain plain pasta, carrot sticks with hummus, grapes, and slice of cheddar cheese
- Egg salad sandwich, tomato slices, cottage cheese and pineapple rings

❹ **Step 4. Multitask preparation time.** The time required to prepare a meal after a long day can be a major barrier to cooking when it's much easier to get takeout or go for fast food. Make it simple by choosing easy-to-prepare meals that your kids can help put together. Prep as much as possible in advance, even considering spending a few hours on the weekend to prep for the week, and then simply freeze and reheat. Most proteins, casseroles, soups, cooked beans, grains, and cooked potatoes are amenable to freezing and reheating. For best results, make sure foods cool completely, then freeze them tightly in an airtight container or freezer bag. When reheating, plan to cook frozen foods an additional 15 minutes or so from their usual cook times. Frozen meals can typically be stored in the freezer for 2 to 3 months.

❺ **Step 5. Implement mealtime rules.** We recommend the following guidelines, or your own variations of them, to not only help family meals be easy and pleasant but also reinforce healthful habits, manners, and responsibility for the children:

- Our family meals are a screen-free event. We will avoid phones, TV, and other distractions while eating.
- We will sit at the table together and, regardless of whether anyone eats, strive toward 20 minutes seated together, if possible.
- We will not hover, badger, micromanage, complain, or otherwise contribute to making mealtimes together an unpleasant experience.
- We will excuse ourselves prior to leaving the table.
- Everyone will play some age-appropriate role in helping to prepare or clean up dinner. (Table 5.1 offers several examples of how family members of different ages can play their part.)

Table 5.1. Prep, Cook, and Clean Up: Age-Appropriate Responsibilities and Opportunities

Having kids involved in the kitchen extends beyond helping to cook. By providing them opportunities to assist, you help them develop life skills, teamwork, and responsibility. Plus, it can make your job a little bit easier. The following table provides examples of ways kids can help in the kitchen:

Age/Stage	How to Help
Toddler (1–3 years)	• Wipe counters. • Place napkins on the table. • Turn on the dishwasher.
Preschool (3–5 years)	• Set the table. • Place dirty dishes on the counter. • Throw away trash. • Wash produce. • Operate food processor. • Help load/unload the dishwasher. • Count ingredients.
School (5–12 years)	• Help make meals. • Carry groceries in from the car. • Put dishes in the dishwasher. • Sweep. • Pour drinks. • Pack lunch. • Take out the garbage.
Teen (12–17 years)	• Put away groceries. • Clean fruits and vegetables and store in plastic containers. • Put dishes away. • Empty the pantry. • Clean the refrigerator. • Plan the menu. • Prepare meals.

Even if you are already participating in all of the 5 steps, family meals with a selective eater can be a source of stress for many families. The good news is that just because a child has picky preferences now doesn't mean it always has to be that way. In fact, hopefully you have already seen some significant changes in your child's willingness to try new foods over the past 4 weeks. But, remember, transforming eating preferences is a process. Remember to

- **Keep mealtimes relaxing and enjoyable.** Have fun together as a family and don't dwell on the food. If the child refuses the meal, don't make a big deal out of it. Remember your "picky-free parenting" rules from week 1.

- **Choose at least one food you know your child will like.** This way, you not only ensure your child will eat something during the meal but also show your child you do care about his preferences when planning meals.

- **Engage your child in meal preparation and cooking.** For example, while grocery shopping, ask your child to pick out one fruit or vegetable that he would like to try at dinner that night. Let the kids have a say in what the meal will be, within certain limits. Invite your children into the kitchen to help prepare the meal.

- **Use "food bridges."** Once a food is accepted, find similarly colored, flavored, or textured food bridges to expand the variety of foods a child will eat. For example, if a child likes pumpkin pie, try mashed sweet potatoes and then mashed carrots. (More on this in our bridging experiment [Try It Out: A Bridging Game].)

- **Spice it up.** Do your best to make the foods look and taste good. It sounds simple enough, but ask around and you'll quickly find people permanently turned off to fresh fish after childhood meals of unappetizing frozen fish sticks, or others unwilling to try fresh, steamed vegetables after too many dinners forced to eat the limp and overcooked kind. Taste is the strongest predictor of whether a child will continue to eat a food she tried. If it is perceived as "gross," it will be difficult to encourage the child to give it another try. Help make food taste delicious by adding herbs and spices to simple meals, collect delicious and healthy recipes (like the ones here!), and learn cooking basics, including how to improvise to make the food taste just right for your family's taste buds.

■ **Offer it often.** Children learn to like what's familiar to them. Just because a child rejects a food once, don't label it "rejected." Instead, continue to reintroduce it and expect that it will take about 15 times before the child will accept it. Rather than pressuring a child to take one bite to get the taste exposure, use other strategies, such as making the food look irresistible. Do this by creating a plate full of color or arranging foods to make a fun shape, by including ingredients that fill the room with a pleasant aroma when cooked (such as ginger, caramelized onions, home-made bread, or cinnamon and honey, such as in our Melting Apples recipe on page 153), or by combining it with a favorite food. To minimize food waste, offer the food in small amounts and wait at least a week or two before reintroducing the same food.

If your kids continue to refuse healthy foods, it's not worth a fight. Hold firm on refusing to make just-for-kids foods and then patiently continue to practice some of the strategies to undo picky eating (review our 10 Rules of Picky-Free Parenting section in Chapter 1 on page 13 if you need a refresher) while also providing a multivitamin in the meantime, if you are feeling very concerned your child may be missing out on needed vitamins and minerals. All along, engage your child's pediatrician to help you troubleshoot and support you on your Picky Eater Project adventure.

TRY IT OUT

A Bridging Game

Kids prefer to eat foods that have a similar taste or texture as foods they already like. Realizing this can help you expand your child's repertoire of foods without a mealtime battle through the use of bridging. Put this to work with our bridging exercise.

Step 1. Think of your child's top 5 favorite foods.

Step 2. For each food you listed, think of a food very similar in taste or texture to that food.

Step 3. Offer your child the "new" food.

Step 4. For each new food offered, think of a different food very similar in taste or texture.

Step 5. Offer your child the "new new" food.

Step 6. Repeat with another set of your child's most preferred foods.

For example,

Top Food	Potential "New" Food	Potential "New New" Food
French fries	Sweet potato fries	Zucchini fries
Chicken nuggets	Fish nuggets	Crispy baked fish
Hamburger	Salmon burger	Grilled salmon sandwich
Cheese pizza	Cheese pizza with whole-grain crust	Cheese pizza with whole-grain crust and homemade (real tomato) pizza sauce

YOUR PICKY EATER PROJECT—WEEK 5

Family Mini-feast

Project To-dos Checklist

☐ Create a weekly meal plan for your family at the beginning of the week, and make an effort to stick to it.

☐ Eat at least 3 family meals together or, at a minimum, the goal number of meals together you established for your family at the beginning of the week.

☐ At each meal, ask each family member the favorite and least favorite part of his or her day.

Project Check-in

❶ Welcome to week 5. What is one thing you've accomplished so far that you are really proud of? What really clicked for you and your family between last week and this week? What do you hope will happen before the Picky Eater Project concludes?

❷ How well did you practice your "picky-free parenting" rules this week?

❸ On a scale of 1 to 10 (1 being the least successful; 10 being the most), how successful was your concerted effort to eat more family meals together? What would make it easier on you to be able to be consistent?

Resources

- Berge JM, Rowley S, Trofholz A, et al. Childhood obesity and interpersonal dynamics during family meals. *Pediatrics.* 2014;134(5):923–932

- Eisenberg ME, Olson RE, Neumark-Sztainer D, Story M, Bearinger LH. Correlations between family meals and psychosocial well-being among adolescents. *Arch Pediatr Adolesc Med.* 2004;158(8):792–796

- Hammons AJ, Fiese BH. Is frequency of shared family meals related to the nutritional health of children and adolescents? *Pediatrics.* 2011;127(6):e1565–e1574

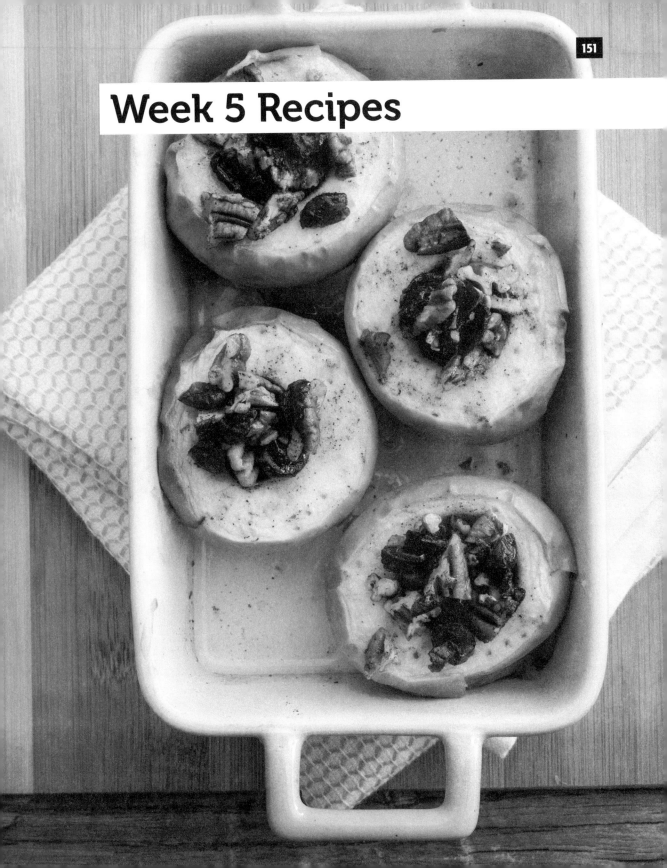

Week 5 Recipes

Melting Apples

Hands-on time: 20 minutes
Total time: 1 hour, 20 minutes
Makes: 4 servings

When you bake apples, the skin more or less keeps its shape, but the inside gets nice and tender, so you can spoon out delicious bites of melted apple. In this recipe, we've sprinkled the apples with cinnamon and stuffed them with a mixture of dried fruit and nuts. Add a different spice or change the filling to create your own variation.

Kitchen Gear

Cutting board

Small bowl

Sharp knife

Measuring cup

Measuring spoons

Melon baller or spoon

Fork

Small baking dish or muffin pan

Pot holder

Ingredients

4 Granny Smith or other tart apples, top third of the apple cut off

¼ cup dried fruit like raisins, dried cranberries, currants, or chopped dried apricots or prunes

¼ cup coarsely chopped lightly roasted nuts like walnuts or pecans

1 tablespoon maple syrup, brown sugar, or honey (sweetener)

½ teaspoon ground cinnamon

¼ cup water

Instructions

1. Turn the oven on and set it to 375 degrees Fahrenheit.

2. Place the apples on a cutting board and remove the top two-thirds of the core by using a melon baller or spoon.

3. Lightly prick the top of the sides of the apple with a fork (this prevents the apples from splitting).

4. Put the dried fruit, nuts, sweetener, and cinnamon in a small bowl. Divide the mixture into 4 parts and stuff it inside the apples.

5. Put the water in the baking dish. Place the apples on top of the water, standing up. Carefully put the baking dish in the oven and bake until the apples are soft, about 1 hour.

6. Serve right away or cover and refrigerate up to 2 days.

Melting Apples *(cont)*

Personalize It

- Taste test the different types of dried fruit and nuts to decide which you'd like to add to your recipe.

- Make baked pears by substituting pears for the apples.

- Substitute dried ginger or nutmeg for the cinnamon.

Kids in the Kitchen

- Let your child pick which dried fruit and nuts to add.

- Let your child measure the dried fruit and nuts.

- Show your child how to core the apple.

Fajitas

Hands-on time: 35 minutes
Total time: 45 minutes (not including marinating time)
Makes: 6 servings

This is a popular Mexican dish that involves grilled beef, shrimp, or chicken in tortillas, often combined with grilled onions and peppers. With all the yummy add-your-own toppings, it makes a meal in itself. Also, it's delicious when served with spicy black bean salad.

Marinate the meat long enough to make it tender and flavorful, but not so long that the acid in the marinade starts to make the meat mushy.

Kitchen Gear

Cutting board

Knife

Measuring cup

Measuring spoons

Medium-sized shallow
  glass or ceramic bowl

Skillet

Heatproof plate

Aluminum foil

Ingredients

1 pound boneless, skinless chicken or turkey breasts, trimmed of
  fat and cut into thin strips

¼ large red onion, coarsely chopped

½ cup homemade or store-bought salsa

¼ cup chopped fresh cilantro leaves

¼ cup fresh lime juice

¼ cup orange juice

¼ to ½ teaspoon crushed red pepper flakes

1 tablespoon vegetable or olive oil

2 red onions, thinly sliced

2 red or yellow bell peppers, cored, seeded, and thinly sliced

8 to 12 flour tortillas

For Serving the Fajitas

Freshly chopped cilantro

Plain yogurt

1 ripe avocado, thinly sliced

Salsa, store-bought or homemade

Fajitas *(cont)*

Instructions

1. Place the uncooked chicken strips in the bowl and add the onion, salsa, cilantro, lime juice, orange juice, and red pepper flakes. Cover and refrigerate at least 1 hour and no more than 4 hours.

2. Turn the oven on and set it to 250 degrees Fahrenheit.

3. Place the skillet on the stove and turn the heat to medium. When it is hot, carefully add half the oil. Add the onions and peppers and cook until the vegetables begin to soften and brown, 10 to 15 minutes. Move the vegetables to the heatproof plate and put in the oven to keep warm.

4. Wrap the tortillas in aluminum foil and put them on an oven rack to heat until ready to use.

5. Using the same skillet you cooked the vegetables in, turn the heat to high. Add the remaining 1½ teaspoons oil. Add the marinated chicken strips. Cook until they have browned, about 2 to 3 minutes, turning once.

6. Carefully remove the plate with the peppers from the oven. Move the peppers to one side and add the chicken tenders.

7. Serve, buffet style, with the cilantro, yogurt, avocado, and salsa in separate bowls, allowing all to assemble their own fajita.

Personalize It

Let your child choose which ingredients he'd like to top his fajitas with: cilantro, yogurt, avocado, and salsa or other toppings from your fridge.

Kids in the Kitchen

- Let your child measure and add each ingredient for the meat marinade.

- Have her wrap the tortillas in foil.

- Show your child how to turn the chicken strips while they are cooking in the skillet.

Fish Tacos

Hands-on time: 45 minutes
Total time: 45 minutes
Makes: 4 servings

There are lots of ingredients to prepare, but this isn't a hard recipe to make, and the tacos are so good. If you don't have (or like) all the taco bar fixings, just use what you do!

Kitchen Gear	**Ingredients**
Clean dish towel	2 tablespoons vegetable or olive oil
Fork	1 teaspoon ground cumin
Measuring spoons	1 teaspoon chili powder
Sharp knife	¼ teaspoon salt
Cutting board	1 garlic clove peeled and minced, or put through a garlic press
Measuring cup	1½ pound halibut fillets (or another firm white fish)
Medium bowl or pie plate	6 (6-inch) corn tortillas
Medium-sized pan	½ onion, finely chopped
Large nonstick pan	1 cup chopped fresh tomato
Spatula	1 cup diced avocado
	½ cup fresh cilantro leaves
	Lime wedges
	Hot sauce
	Plain Greek yogurt

Instructions

1. Mix the oil, spices, salt, and garlic in a bowl.

2. Cut the fish into 1-inch strips, place them in the bowl or pie plate, and use clean fingers to coat them with the spice mixture. Set the bowl aside. Wash your hands.

3. Place the medium-sized pan over medium heat and when it is hot, add the tortillas one at a time. Cook for about 30 seconds and then wrap in a clean dish towel to keep warm.

4. Place the large nonstick pan on the stove and turn the heat to medium-high. Place the fish in the hot pan and cook for 3 minutes; then use the spatula to flip the pieces over. Cook on the other side until the fish breaks easily into flakes when you poke it with a fork, around 2 minutes.

5. Give each person 2 tortillas and let all assemble the tacos with whatever ingredients they like.

Fish Tacos *(cont)*

Personalize It

Prepare small bowls of the following additions for before, during, or after cooking:

- Cabbage (purple or green)
- Kale
- Radish
- Thinly sliced red onion

Kids in the Kitchen

- Let your child coat the fish with the spice mixture using his clean fingers.
- Have your child flip the tortilla halfway through cook time while they are being warmed using tongs.
- Using a spatula, teach your child how to flip the fish.
- Let your child assemble the tacos, allowing him to choose whatever toppings/add-ons he'd like.

Sweet Potato Bar

Hands-on time: 20 minutes
Total time: 1 hour, 20 minutes
Makes: 4 servings

Baked sweet potatoes are great all on their own or as receptacles for other flavors. Try any of our suggestions or add your own!

—Recipe by Catherine Newman

Kitchen Gear

Fork

Baking Sheet

Pot holder

Cutting Board

Sharp knife

Ingredients

4 Idaho or sweet potatoes

Your choice of toppings

Instructions

1. Turn the oven on and set it to 450 degrees Fahrenheit.

2. Using the tines of the fork, plunge it into each potato a few times to make a few holes.

3. Carefully put the potatoes directly on the rack in the oven. Place a baking sheet on a lower rack (this is to catch any oozy drips). Bake until tender when pushed down, about 1 hour.

4. Carefully, using a pot holder, put the potatoes on the cutting board and cut in half. Squeeze both ends to make the potato open. Serve right away with little bowls of condiments.

Personalize It

- Butter or olive oil and kosher salt

- Chopped fresh basil or cilantro leaves

- Grated cheddar, Monterey Jack, Parmesan, feta, or goat cheese

- Plain yogurt, Greek or traditional

- Lemon or lime quarters, for squeezing

- A sprinkle of ground spice, including cinnamon, curry, garam masala, nutmeg, ginger, or cardamom

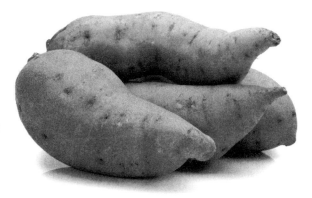

Sweet Potato Bar *(cont)*

Kids in the Kitchen

- Using child-safe scissors or her hands, your child can cut or tear the fresh basil or cilantro leaves into small pieces.

- Have your child grate her own cheese, or crumble with her fingers.

- Have your child squeeze the lemons and limes. Taste test each to see if she can taste the difference!

- Teach your child how to measure the spices using measuring spoons.

Vegetable Chili

Hands-on time: 40 minutes
Total time: 1 hour, 40 minutes
Makes: 6 to 8 servings

Chili can sometimes be spicy, but this recipe is designed to be mild. If you want to go for the burn, add the extra spices listed in the Ingredients section or fresh or dried chili peppers. You can use lots of different vegetables, but we especially like silky sweet butternut squash or eggplant, which adds a kind of meatiness. Be absolutely sure you cook both until they are very soft!

Kitchen Gear

Can opener

Measuring spoons

Sharp knife

Cutting board

Measuring cups

Colander or strainer

Large heavy-bottomed
  pot with lid

Large spoon

Pot holder

Ingredients

2 teaspoons olive or vegetable oil

1 large onion, chopped

3 garlic cloves, peeled, and minced or chopped

3 cups peeled and diced butternut squash or eggplant

2 red, orange, or yellow bell peppers, cored, seeded, and diced

2 to 4 tablespoons chili powder (or more to taste)

1 to 1½ teaspoons dried oregano

1 to 2 teaspoons ground cumin (or more to taste)

1 teaspoon crushed red pepper flakes (if you like it spicy)

¼ to ½ teaspoon cayenne pepper (if you like it spicy)

¼ cup water (if you need it)

4 cups cooked or canned dark red kidney beans, drained and rinsed

2 cups cooked or canned black beans, drained and rinsed

2 (28-ounce) cans diced tomatoes, including the juice

2 small or 1 large zucchini, diced

Vegetable Chili *(cont)*

Instructions

1. Place the pot on the stove and turn the heat to medium. When it is hot, carefully add the oil.

2. Add the onion, garlic, butternut squash, bell peppers, chili powder, oregano, cumin, and red pepper flakes and cayenne (if you like it spicy) and cook on low heat until the vegetables have softened, about 20 minutes. Stir from time to time. If it looks dry, add the water.

3. Add the beans and tomatoes and cook covered, stirring occasionally, for 30 minutes.

4. Add the zucchini and cook uncovered until the zucchini is tender, about 20 minutes.

5. Serve right away, or cover and refrigerate up to 3 days.

Personalize It

- Make it spicy using the optional foods and spices in the ingredients.
- Add 2 cups of fresh or frozen corn kernels.

Kids in the Kitchen

Try doing a chili taste test with your kids to determine how spicy you'd like your chili. Have your child try the chili before adding spice and then after adding spice: Do you want to make it spicier?

CHAPTER 6

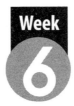

It Takes a Village

"It takes a whole village
to raise a child."

— African Proverb

Mission
Gather support from peers, school, grandparents,
and other influential people in your child's life.

Strategy
Engage outside influencers in your Picky Eater Project.

Measurement
Number of successful food or mealtime experiences
with nonparent influencers.

Marlo and Corey learned of the powerful influence of "the village" in helping to raise more adventurous eaters during an impromptu dinner at their house with the neighbors (who were privy to the Picky Eater Project underway next door). Marlo and Corey prepared steak, rice, and caprese, a tomato and mozzarella salad. Their neighbors brought steamed mussels and a variety of fresh vegetables and fruits, among them green grapes, oranges, spicy green peppers, carrots, heirloom tomatoes, and grape tomatoes. The kids had just gotten home from swimming practice and were very hungry. The timing was somewhat strategic, as hungry kids—and adults—are generally more willing to eat whatever is placed in front of them.

The youngest neighbor turned out to have a very adventurous palate. As soon as the food was set out, she propped herself at the kitchen island and started snacking on the mussels, carrots, and tomatoes, and even took a bite of the spicy pepper. At first, the older kids didn't pay much attention. Hunter started trolling through the pantry looking for bread, and Marlo gently redirected him to choose from the foods that were available in the kitchen as appetizers. Hunter was hungry so he chose the green grapes but also tried a grape tomato and carrots, both of which he liked.

A New Favorite Food Realized

After noticing his friend eating the mussels, Hunter seemed intrigued. He kept walking by and eyeing them. He said he was afraid to eat the mussels because they might make him throw up. He started sniffing them. He then went to Corey and asked him what he thought about "that weird-looking food over there. What is it made of?" He dared Brooke and his other friend to try one but they refused. He asked Corey what it tasted like, then picked one up and smelled it, and eventually licked it. Marlo, who during this whole scenario was pretending not to notice, stopped herself from cajoling Hunter into trying a mussel. She couldn't believe what happened next; Hunter took the mussel out of the shell and popped it in his mouth. Chewed. Swallowed. And then said it was delicious and he really liked it.

That was enough for his more reluctant friend to try the mussels. And then, Brooke, who is the more cautious and picky of the two, noticed everyone else was trying them, so she came over and tried one herself. She said it was actually pretty good, but "tasted odd, like the texture of bubblegum," and liked how salty it tasted. But one was enough for her. Hunter ate several more and at the end of the night declared mussels to be his new favorite food.

As everyone sat down for dinner, Marlo and Corey implemented the one-meal rule. Brooke and Hunter would not be getting a separate meal tonight. The kids didn't seem to mind and continued to eat their favorite parts of the dinner with their friends (mostly the steak and white rice). They didn't eat or even try everything on their plates, and that was OK.

Marlo and Corey felt the meal was a big success, that clearly peer influence—more than parental—had made a tremendous effect on Hunter's and, subsequently, Brooke's interest in trying the foods, and they expressed hope that some of this newfound willingness to try a new food would carry over into their own regular family meals.

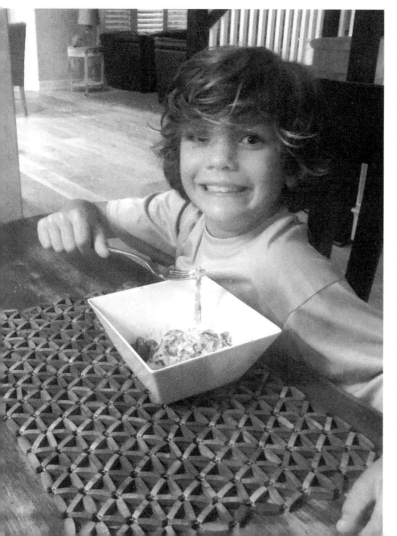

As Marlo and Corey realized, and at this point in your own Picky Eater Project you likely have too, this plan to reform selective eating preferences works best with buy-in and support from other important people in your child's life. From neighbors, friends, and roommates to parents, stepparents, siblings, and grandparents—everyone has a very important role to play. It takes a village to undo picky eating. And with the right supports, this plan can also undo a village of picky eaters! This week we will work on the social supports to help everyone own the change.

Leaning on the Village to Undo Picky Eating

The village consists of the many influential people in your child's life, including parents and stepparents, grandparents, siblings, peers, schools and teachers, babysitters and other caretakers, and neighbors. When it comes to eating preferences, the most important influencer is the nutritional gatekeeper, typically a parent who does most of the grocery shopping and meal preparation. But the influences of others, especially peers, schools, and grandparents, add up quickly.

Modeling the Way

Children may learn to like foods they see their parents, peers, and other important people in their lives eat. The most powerful models are the people children see as similar to themselves (peers) or as particularly powerful (older peers and siblings and parents). In one study, toddlers put food in their mouths more readily when they were following the example of their mother compared with a stranger. In another study, younger siblings got up the courage to try the generally aversive-tasting chili peppers when they watched older family members eat them. It goes without saying that one of the most powerful strategies you can apply to raising healthy eaters is to model healthy eating for them and expose them to healthy models, including yourselves, peers, family members, and other people who your children admire.

The Power of Peers

Just as parental modeling affects what kids choose to eat, so does peer modeling. As kids grow up, peers play an increasingly important role in shaping attitudes, preferences, and behaviors. Peers reinforce—pay attention to, praise, criticize, or share—one another's behaviors. This reinforcement—whether positive or negative—goes a long way in shaping a child's behavior. A child who spends time at a friend's house where the norm is to eat unfamiliar snacks is more likely to try those snacks if he sees his friend enjoying them. The opposite, of course, is also true. A child who likes vegetables but gets made fun of by his friends for eating them is less likely to want to continue to eat vegetables.

Highly regarded older peers, such as siblings, mentors, and babysitters, tend to play a particularly important role in influencing a child's preferences. Basically 4 "ingredients" are required for modeling experiences to make an impression on a child.

❶ Noticing what is going on

❷ Remembering the event

❸ Reproducing the behavior

❹ Imitating the behavior

You don't have to leave it to luck whether any or all of these ingredients are present. Set the stage. When something big is going to happen that you want your child to model (eg, trying an unfamiliar or previously rejected food), make sure you're prepared to maximize the chances your child will take note.

- **Minimize distractions.** For example, if you're going to be eating a family meal together with a lot of vegetables and a child's best friend (who also happens to be a vegetable lover) as a guest, make sure during dinner the TV and cell phones are off, no one's rushing to go anywhere or finish quickly, and your child is seated in close proximity to his friend. This makes it more likely that your child will notice his friend's behavior and want to imitate it.

- **Make the occasion worth remembering.** Pair the desired activity (in this case, eating a new food) with something fun or some memorable jingle or experience. Fast-food restaurants and food marketers do a great job at thinking up catchy gimmicks that stick. It could be as simple as thinking of wacky names for the vegetables you're eating at dinner, such as X-ray Vision Carrots and Power Peas, names studies from Cornell Food and Brand Lab have shown to work in increasing intake in younger kids.

- **Choose reproducible activities.** An outing to a new exotic restaurant could be a way to encourage a child to try something new, but if the food will never be available at home, the experience is unlikely to stick in expanding a child's food preferences. Rather, you might try a new easy-to-make recipe that pairs a child's favorite food with a new food. Practice the strategy of pairing to broaden your child's food repertoire with our pairing experiment and score sheet (Try It Out: A Pairing Adventure).

- **Highlight major motivators.** What really makes your child tick? Is it a favorite TV character, spending time with a best friend, performing well at a sport, getting good grades? Connect food and nutritional offerings and education with things that are important to your child. For example, if your child loves soccer, remind her that making healthy nutritional choices will help her have the energy and focus to play better. If your son is a star student, he might be interested to know that kids who eat a healthy breakfast perform better on tests. While optimizing health is important to parents, it's often not a major motivator for kids and teens.

TRY IT OUT

A Pairing Adventure

You can help your child like unfamiliar foods with tastes your child innately dislikes (sour and bitter) by pairing them with familiar foods the child innately prefers (sweet and salty). For example, grapefruit (sour) paired with a drizzle of honey (sweet) is more likely to be accepted than the grapefruit alone. Fresh cranberries (tart) taste best when boiled with a little bit of sugar (sweet). Broccoli (bitter) with grated cheese (salty) could be a way to introduce broccoli into your child's list of tolerable foods. Or you could try pairing vegetables with sauces, such as sweet barbeque or salty soy (go with the low-sodium version to retain the salty flavor). While it's best to minimize a lot of extra added salt and sugar, pairing small amounts of these tastes with new foods helps children become more willing to try and ultimately like new foods.

Put this notion of pairing to practice with your kids and their friends with this pairing experiment.

❶ Ask your child to invite 2–3 of his best friends over for a pairing party. Together with the kids cut up a variety of raw vegetables, such as carrots, cucumbers, celery, broccoli, cauliflower, black olives, radishes, jicama, various-colored peppers, and tomatoes. Also, cut up a variety of fresh fruits, such as apples, pears, grapes, and strawberries.

❷ Then, with the kids, make a few of these dips.

- White Bean Dip (For recipe, see page 181.)
- Guacamole (See page 184.)
- Classic Hummus (See Chapter 3, page 85.)
- Date Nut Cream Cheese (See page 185.)
- Cucumber Tsatziki (See page 183.)
- Homemade Peanut Butter (See page 186.)

❸ Ask each child to choose one of each of the vegetables and fruits, try each, and score them on a scale of 1 (no thanks!) to 10 (delicious!).

❹ Have them dip each of the vegetables and fruits into any of the various dips and score them again on a scale of 1 (no thanks!) to 10 (delicious!). Use the score sheet that follows to record their scores.

❺ Next, go through each vegetable and fruit and ask the kids if their score of the food changed when they tried it with the dip. If so, ask them why they thought that happened.

❻ Compare the responses of each of the kids.

❼ Ask each child to identify a favorite vegetable, fruit, and dip.

❽ Print out the favorite dip recipe for your child's friend to take home.

A Pairing Adventure Score Sheet (Include a score of 1–10 in each box.)

Fruit/Vegetable	Alone	White Bean Dip	Classic Hummus	Cucumber Tsatziki	Guacamole	Date Nut Cream Cheese	Homemade Peanut Butter	Total Score (The fruits and vegetables with the highest scores are your favorites!)
Carrots								
Cucumber								
Celery								
Broccoli								
Cauliflower								
Black olives								
Radishes								
Jicama								
Peppers								
Tomatoes								
Apples								
Pears								
Grapes								
Strawberries								
Other								
Total Score (The dips with the highest scores are your favorites!)								

Eating Healthy at School

School is a powerful influencer in a child's life. Clocking in nearly 40 hours a week, many kids eat breakfast, lunch, and snacks at school. This offers a big opportunity for a child to expand eating preferences.

Over the past several years, food offered at schools has generally gotten much healthier, with federal regulation requiring schools to

- Increase fruits and vegetables served and require children to select a fruit, a vegetable, or both as part of school lunch or breakfast.

- Emphasize whole grains at meals.

- Limit calories and sodium in school breakfast, lunch, and snacks.

- Eliminate trans fat, also known as partially hydrogenated oil.

- Offer snacks that have whole grains, a fruit, a vegetable, a dairy product, or protein-rich food as the first ingredient.

While the school lunch is certainly easier—and with the increasingly healthy school lunch offerings, often healthier—sending your kids to school with a lunch at least a couple of times per week gives you an excellent opportunity to help shape their eating habits. Of course, it's a delicate balance. The decision between what you would like your child to eat versus what you think she will actually consume influences your choices. Should you put in the carrots you know she will reject just so she's exposed to the vegetables? How about her favorite chocolate chip cookies simply because you know how happy it will make her? Without you there looking over your kids' shoulders and supervising intake, lunchtime and snack time at school offers kids an opportunity to exert some control over food choices and put into practice what you've been teaching them at home. They may choose to trash, barter, or eat your carefully planned meal. Box 6.1 offers some tips on packing a lunch for your child.

Box 6.1. Packed Lunch Tips and Ideas

When helping your child pack a lunch (note: we say *helping* your child rather than *packing your child a lunch* because as young as preschool, kids can play a very active role in making lunch), keep the following tips in mind:

Involve your child. The best way to ensure your kids will actually eat the food you put in their lunch box is to give them some control of what goes in there. Even the pickiest eaters enjoy some healthy foods. Be sure to include at least one healthy item your child loves. And next time you head out to the grocery store, ask for your kids' input into what *healthy food* they'd like to have in their lunch boxes. The mere exercise of helping them sort through their favorites will help them learn what types of foods are healthy for their bodies and which ones are less healthy.

Aim for balance. Try to include something from each of the major food groups—a whole grain; a protein-containing food, such as meat, beans, or legumes; a fruit; a vegetable; and a dairy product or another calcium-containing food—in your child's lunch box every day. Even if she chooses not to eat it all, your child will start to pick up on what a balanced meal includes.

Increase exposure to healthy foods. Use lunchtime as an opportunity to expose your children to a small amount of a previously rejected food. Even if they choose not to eat, mere exposure may help increase the chances they'll appreciate it in the future. As we have mentioned a few times—but definitely worth repeating—it often takes 15 to 20 tries for a child to accept a previously rejected food.

Teach portion control. Preparing lunch gives you a perfect opportunity to pay attention to portion control. Use plastic bags, attempt to measure out standard portions, and include some inherently portion-controlled items for the lunch box, such as an apple or string cheese.

Make eating healthy fun. Kids, especially preschool- and elementary-aged children, love foods that are packaged in a fun way. Perhaps your child will be more likely to eat the baby carrots if you package them in a funnily decorated baggy. Or maybe your child will totally reject celery and raisins if offered separately, but when they're presented as "ants on a log" (celery with peanut butter and raisins), she might gobble it up. Just be careful to avoid marketing tricks in which junk foods are packaged with your child's favorite characters (eg, SpongeBob fruit snacks). This just helps your child love the sugary stuff even more.

Here are some easy-to-make lunch ideas that follow the above suggestions and could help your children expand their food preferences.

- Peanut butter (no sugar added) and sliced banana sandwich on whole-grain bread cut into quarters. Try the Homemade Peanut Butter recipe on page 186. Include a few baby carrots and dried fruit.

- Turkey sandwich with hummus and tomato on whole-grain bread. Add string cheese, crackers, an apple, and a couple of fig bars.

- Try last night's leftovers. Don't forget to include a plastic fork/spoon/knife (if needed) and an ice pack to keep it cold. Add a few cherry tomatoes, a hard-boiled egg, and some applesauce.

- California rolls with edamame and red grapes.

As kids enter the upper elementary school grades, we suggest transitioning the job of preparing lunch to them. Share with them the lunch box requirement of balance and let them decide what goes in. Before transitioning the responsibility, you could give them a quick lesson on the things you consider when making a lunch, such as going for high-fiber whole grain rather than the highly processed white version, leaner meats, and fruits and vegetables of different colors. Initially, you might inspect to make sure lunch doesn't include just several cookies and a soda (although by now, you probably don't have these in the house!), but eventually, you might want to slowly transition to trusting their choices and periodically giving a surprise inspection.

Remember, for the most part, kids will have available to them only items they can find in the house. This offers you a good opportunity to double-check whether you're maximizing access to healthy foods and minimizing access to the more highly processed and less healthy versions. Don't forget to also teach your kids to throw in a couple of ice packs to keep perishable foods cold. One study found that by the time kids actually ate their food, more than 90% of lunches contained items that were above a safe temperature, leaving those kids susceptible to food-borne illness.

Grandparents

Grandparents are profoundly important in the lives of children. For many families, they help provide stability, support, and child care. Not to mention they've already raised kids of their own. In most cases, it would be a mistake to shun the help of a loving grandparent. However, without some structure and general guidelines for when your kids are with their grandparents, you might find that an influential, firm-minded grandparent could swiftly and completely undo the progress you've made over the past few weeks. On the other hand, a supportive grandparent could further reinforce and help solidify your progress. This is especially the case when grandparents live nearby and spend a lot of time with the children in a caretaking role.

We suggest the following strategies when trying to help a grandparent get on board with your new plan:

- Always try to show your appreciation and gratitude to grandparents, especially when they go out of their way to help out or go along with your requests.

- Share any concerns in a transparent and open manner. That is, set up a time in advance to have a conversation about your child's health. Identify shared values (you both want your child to be happy and healthy) and try to strategize ways together to help your child be happy and healthy. If you feel undermined or ignored, say that. For example, "I feel undermined when you take my child to get ice cream after school when you know I am having trouble with him eating dinner due to snacking before we eat. I know we both want what is best for him. Will you work with me to come up with a plan to help him develop better eating habits?"

- You set the rules at your house, but consider letting Grandma set the rules at her house (this may work best when your kids do not spend a lot of time at their grandparents' homes). Kids are place specific. They understand that different places may have different rules. To the best extent possible, create a situation in which most mealtimes occur in your home and where other household members follow along with your plan.

- When watching the kids at your house, make it easy for the grandparents to follow your "picky-free parenting" rules.

- Explain the rationale for why you do what you do.

- Choose your battles wisely.

- Enlist the help of others who the grandparents respect and trust, such as your child's pediatrician, other family members, or family friends.

- Tolerate some spoiling.

- Create opportunities for kids and their grandparents to be healthy and active together. For example, they might take a cooking class, garden, go hiking or bike riding, or learn a new sport together.

Overall, the main goal of this week is to gather as much support as possible from peers, school, grandparents, and other people who are influential in your child's life. At the same time, appreciate that many influences will be difficult, if not impossible, to control. Sometimes the best approach is doing everything you can to help raise healthy, well-adjusted children, and trust that even though some things are out of your control, you have taught your children how to make good choices—and eventually they will do so—even when you are not there looking over their shoulder.

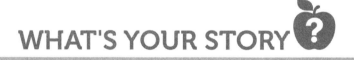

WHAT'S YOUR STORY

How involved are your child's grandparents in your Picky Eater Project? Are they generally supportive or not so much? What specific steps might you take to gain their support?

YOUR PICKY EATER PROJECT—WEEK 6

It Takes a Village

Project To-dos Checklist

☐ Invite one of your child's friends over to your house for dinner and prepare a food that you know your child's friend likes but that maybe your child would typically not try. What happened? Did your child try the food?

☐ Arrange for your child to go over to a friend's house for dinner. In advance, speak with the friend's parents to see if they might be willing to offer a new food that their child loves but perhaps your child has never tried before. Ask the parents for a recap of what happened.

☐ Together with your child and a couple of his or her friends, try out the pairing experiment (see Try It Out: A Pairing Adventure on pages 170–171).

☐ List 3 ways you are creating a healthy, adventurous food environment for your family. In addition, come up with 3 ways you could make small, doable changes to further support your children and other family members making healthy choices.

Project Check-in

❶ As you wrap up week 6, you are nearing the end of your Picky Eater Project. What did you hope to gain from the project that you haven't already? Consider making that a focus for next week.

❷ Who did you identify as your biggest supporters as you participated in the Picky Eater Project? Who made it more challenging? Acknowledge the supporters.

❸ What experience this week most stuck out to you? Why?

Resources

- Harper LV, Sanders KM. The effect of adults' eating on young children's acceptance of unfamiliar foods. *J Exp Child Psychol.* 1975;20:206–214
- Rozin P, Schiller D. The nature of a preference for chili pepper by humans. *Motiv Emotion.* 1980;4:77–101

Note: Both of these studies were cited in the excellent reviews Birch LL, Fisher JO. Development of eating behaviors among children and adolescents. *Pediatrics.* 1998;101(3 Pt 2):539–549, and Almansour FD, Sweitzer SJ, Mangess AA, et al. Temperature of foods sent by parents of preschool-aged children. *Pediatrics.* 2011;128(3):519–523.

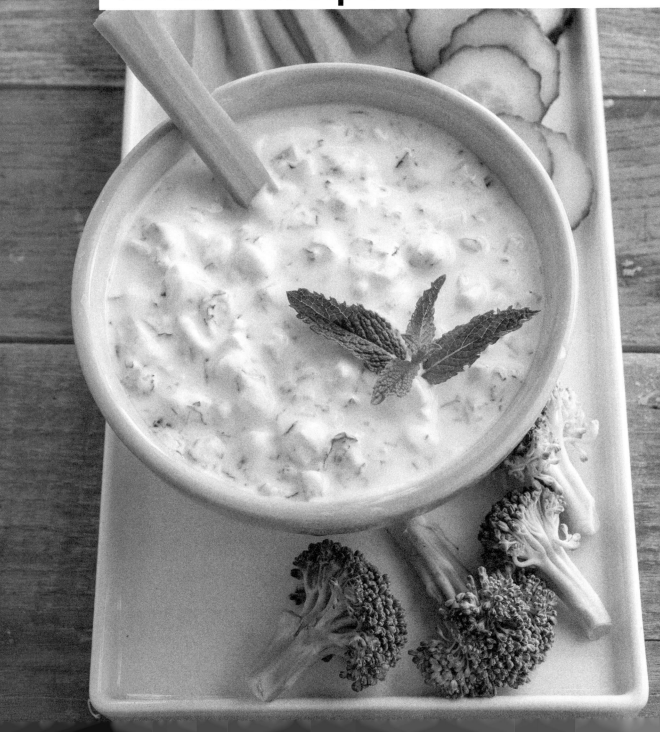

Week 6 Recipes

White Bean Dip

Hands-on time: 15 minutes
Total time: 15 minutes
Makes: 1¼ cups

When you puree beans, they make a rich, creamy dip that's delicious with French bread, pita chips, or raw vegetables. Or use it as a healthier option instead of mayonnaise on a ham or cheese sandwich—it will add lots more flavor and nutrients. For our Classic Hummus recipe, see Chapter 3, page 85.

Kitchen Gear

Cutting board

Can opener

Strainer or colander

Sharp knife

Measuring cup

Measuring spoons

Food processor or fork or
　potato masher

Large spoon

Serving bowl

Ingredients

2 cups cooked or canned white beans, drained and rinsed
　with cold tap water

1 to 2 garlic cloves, peeled, and minced or chopped

¼ cup olive oil

3 tablespoons fresh lemon juice (about 1 lemon)

½ teaspoon kosher salt

¼ teaspoon black pepper

Instructions

1. Pour the white beans, garlic, oil, lemon juice, salt, and pepper in the food processor fitted with a steel blade. Put the top on tightly and process until completely smooth. (If you don't have a food processor, you can mash everything using a fork or potato masher. It won't get as smooth but will definitely be yummy!)

2. Spoon into the serving bowl, cover, and refrigerate at least 1 hour and up to 2 days.

White Bean Dip *(cont)*

Personalize It

Add any of these ingredients to your bean dip for extra flavor!

- 1 to 2 tablespoons chopped fresh basil, parsley, or cilantro leaves, or snipped chives
- 1 teaspoon chopped fresh rosemary
- Grated zest of a lemon
- 1 to 2 tablespoons chopped or pureed olives
- 1 teaspoon chopped jalapeño peppers or hot sauce (if you like it spicy)
- 1 tablespoon pesto

Kids in the Kitchen

- Allow your child to measure and add all ingredients.
- Show your child how to drain and rinse the beans.
- Taste test the personalized add-in ingredients to decide what additional ingredients you'd like in your dip.

Cucumber Tsatziki

Hands-on time: 20 minutes
Total time: 20 minutes
Makes: 4 servings

Tsatziki is a tangy yogurt-based dip from Greece that's great with raw vegetables and pita chips, or spread on tomato sandwiches and burgers, spooned onto a piece of grilled fish, or even mixed into a salad instead of salad dressing.

Kitchen Gear

Peeler

Measuring spoon

Measuring cup

Sharp knife

Cutting board

Small mixing bowl

Ingredients

1 small English cucumber or 1 conventional cucumber, peeled, thinly sliced, and chopped

1 cup plain Greek yogurt (the thickest you can find)

1 garlic clove, peeled, and minced or chopped

¼ cup finely chopped fresh mint leaves, plus extra for garnish (if you like)

¼ teaspoon kosher salt

Instructions

1. Combine the cucumber, yogurt, garlic, mint, and salt in the mixing bowl and mix well.

2. Cover and refrigerate at least 1 hour and up to overnight. Serve garnished with the additional mint if you like.

Kids in the Kitchen

- Teach your child how to properly peel the cucumber.

- Using a plastic knife, have your child carefully thinly slice and chop the cucumber.

- Allow your child to measure and add the remaining ingredients.

Guacamole

Hands-on time: 20 minutes
Total time: 20 minutes
Makes: About 1½ cups

This is the classic, pale-green Mexican dip that makes the most of avocados' creaminess. Serve it with tortilla or pita chips, on Beanie Burgers With Cheese (for recipe, see Chapter 3, page 93), on or in quesadillas, or atop a bowl of chili.

Kitchen Gear	Ingredients
Serving bowl	2 ripe Hass avocadoes
Sharp knife	½ fresh tomato, cored and coarsely chopped
Cutting board	1 scallion, greens and whites, chopped
Measuring spoons	1 heaping tablespoon finely chopped fresh cilantro leaves
Spoon	2 teaspoons fresh lime juice
Small bowl	¼ teaspoon kosher salt
Fork	½ to 1 teaspoon hot sauce (if you like)

Instructions

1. Slice each avocado in half. Remove the pit and set it aside. Use a spoon to scoop out the insides. Put the avocado in the small bowl and using a fork, mash it until it is still a little bit chunky.

2. Add the tomato, scallions, cilantro, lime juice, and salt. Mash a bit more, but keep it chunky (unless you like it smooth). Add the hot sauce, if you prefer.

3. Scoop the guacamole into a serving bowl and serve right away or put the pits in the guacamole (to prevent it from turning dark), cover, and refrigerate up to 4 hours.

Personalize It

- Add more scallions.
- Substitute fresh basil leaves for the cilantro.
- Use lemon juice instead of lime juice.

Kids in the Kitchen

- Have your child scoop out the inside of the avocado.
- Let your child mash the avocado using a fork.
- Let your child squeeze the juice from the lime.

Date Nut Cream Cheese

Hands-on time: 10 minutes
Total time: 10 minutes
Makes: 4 servings

This spread makes a delicious and nutritious filling for anything, from a sandwich to a celery stick.

Kitchen Gear
Measuring spoon

Measuring cup

Sharp knife
   or kitchen scissors

Cutting board

Bowl

Fork

Ingredients
7 dates

4 ounces cream cheese (softened at room temperature)

1 tablespoon buttermilk, plain yogurt, or milk

¼ cup chopped toasted walnuts

Instructions
1. Pit and chop the dates. If you like, you can cut them up with a clean pair of scissors.

2. Put the cream cheese and buttermilk, yogurt, or milk in the bowl and using the fork, mash until it is smooth.

3. Add the dates and walnuts and mash until it is all combined.

4. Serve right away or cover and refrigerate up to 3 days.

Personalize It
- Use ¼ cup raisins, dried cranberries, or currants rather than dates.

- Instead of using walnuts, try using almonds or pecans.

Kids in the Kitchen
- Using scissors, have your child carefully cut the dates.

- Using a fork, have your child mash the mixture.

Homemade Peanut Butter

Hands-on time: 3 minutes
Total time: 3 minutes
Makes: 1 cup, enough for about 8 sandwiches

You'll be amazed how easy it is to make your own peanut butter from whole peanuts. It tastes great because it's so fresh, and it doesn't have any of the added sugar or oil that most store-bought peanut butter contains.

Kitchen Gear

Measuring cup

Measuring spoons

Food processor

Rubber spatula

Spoon

Container with lid

Ingredients

2 cups dry-roasted peanuts

Pinch kosher salt or more to taste (less for salted peanuts, more for unsalted)

Instructions

1. Place the peanuts in the food processor fitted with a steel blade. Put the top on tightly and process until they break down and bunch up into a glob in the food processor bowl, about 1 minute.

2. Stop the food processor, take off the top, and carefully scrape around the inside of the bowl with the spatula. Add the salt, put the top back on, and continue to process, stopping 2 or 3 more times to scrape the bowl, until the peanut butter is smooth, about 1 minute longer.

3. Use a spoon to taste a tiny bit of the peanut butter. If you like it saltier, add a pinch of salt, put the top back on, and turn on the food processor to mix in the salt, about 3 seconds.

4. Use the spatula to scrape the peanut butter into a container with a tight-fitting lid. Cover and refrigerate up to 2 weeks. When you take the peanut butter out of the fridge, it will be a little bit hard and difficult to spread, but it will soften after a few minutes on the counter.

Personalize It

- Add dried spices such as cayenne pepper or cinnamon for a kick.
- Add 1 tablespoon unsweetened jam.

Kids in the Kitchen

- Let your child measure and add the ingredients to the food processor.
- Let your child scrape down the inside of the bowl.

CHAPTER 7

Post–Picky Eater Project: Making It Stick-y

"Motivation is what gets you started.
Habit is what keeps you going."

— Jim Ryun, Author

Mission
Make the changes stick for the long run.

Strategy
Anticipate and plan for challenges and setbacks.

Measurement
Number of relapses met with a productive response.

Zucchini pasta. Mussels. Armenian cucumbers. Pomegranates. Corn pancakes. Fish tacos. While Brooke and Hunter didn't love them all, they were willing to give the new foods a try without coercion, bribery, or deal making (for the most part). Over their Picky Eater Project, Brooke and Hunter racked up an impressive list of new acceptable foods. Mostly through changes to Marlo and Corey's parenting approach, the kids gradually ventured outside their comfort zone. Corey remarked that what affected him the most was how willing Hunter was to try very strange new foods (eg, mussels) when an eager friend was over to try them first. He was also thrilled to find the Zucchini Pasta recipe (see Chapter 4, page 135), which the whole family loved, and was impressed with how easy it became to incorporate more fruits and vegetables into the family meals.

We checked back with the family and how close they came to achieving their goals.

Family Project Reflection

MARLO really wanted the kids to eat a greater variety of healthy foods. She reports she is thrilled with the outcome that they really do try new foods and, a little unbelievably, she reveals that they eat more different and exotic foods than they ever would have previously tried. They do not always love them, but they are more willing to try a taste. She also hoped her kids would learn to like fish more. Hunter eventually acquired a taste for sushi, but both Brooke and Hunter are still "training their taste buds" when it comes to other types of fish.

"I just can't stand the smell!" Brooke explains.

Overall, "It's a relief not to feel like I have to force them to eat anymore," Marlo said.

COREY'S goal was that the whole family eat ONE meal and learn a few easy dinner recipes the whole family would like. While Marlo and Corey do still occasionally end up making a couple of different meals to accommodate everyone's tastes, it occurs a LOT less often—"and it's more like 1 or 2 meals now, rather than 3 or 4. So that's a big improvement!" Corey remarked. Excitingly, the Zucchini Pasta recipe has become a frequent favorite for everyone in the family. If the preparation process of peeling the zucchinis was a little less burdensome, they would eat it even more.

BROOKE'S goal was to flip a pancake without having it smear all over the pan (accomplished!) and be trusted to use not just the microwave but also the oven, stove, and toaster (also accomplished!). Additionally, she learned some pretty cool cooking skills that she gets to put to practice frequently. She's also adopted some of the Picky Eater Project techniques for herself. For instance, she loves to tell the story of the time when she and her friend made pancakes for themselves and Hunter. They asked Hunter if he wanted bananas in them. He said not really, but she included them anyway and he loved it!

HUNTER'S goal was to eat more artichokes. While artichokes were not on the menu for much of the 6 weeks, Hunter didn't mind at all because he tried a whole lot of other foods that he didn't think he'd like but did. Corey noted "instead of Hunter deciding he doesn't like something before he tries it, he now will try it first, then decide if he likes it or not. It's a huge, positive change."

"We really can eat a lot more foods now," Corey and Marlo agreed. Weekend breakfast used to be fried eggs only. The kids wouldn't eat the eggs any other way. But now they will eat all styles of eggs, and Brooke loves to get in the kitchen and help make them. While both kids are still working on cleaning up after themselves when they cook (which is a necessity before Marlo and Corey will let them play a more involved role in cooking on a regular basis) and Marlo and Corey are still working on finding enough dinners that everyone will eat (so they don't feel compelled to make a different one to accommodate the kids), overall they feel that their family mealtimes are much more pleasant, enjoyable, and healthy.

Preschool Picky Eater Project

Christine and Fran noticed similarly remarkable changes with their kids. Four-year-old Andrew now embraces foods he previously shunned. And most notably for Christine and Fran, they all sit down together to one meal. Not once in the 6 weeks did Fran or Christine make a separate dish for either boy. Fran says he is "less stressed and more positive about the food being served, compared [with] the poorly kid-customized meals of the past."

Hopefully over the course of the past 6 weeks you've also seen some notable positive changes at your home, from lower-stress mealtimes to a longer list of "acceptable foods." In fact, now is a great time to look back at your initial goal and check in with how close you were to achieving it, what worked well, and what didn't. The key now is helping those behaviors stick at home and generalize across time, places, and people. Use the final goals check-in (see Project Check-in section on page 197) to see how far you've come.

Picky Eater Project: Going Forward

In this chapter, we will plan for challenges and barriers and put the contingency plans into action. Relapses happen. But how we respond to them determines how much of a lasting effect they will have. Just like any other behavioral change, we need a plan for making it stick. These 10 tips will help turn your Picky Eater Project into a normal daily routine.

❶ **Start small.** While it's tempting to want to go from having the most persistently selective eater in the neighborhood to a food connoisseur, the reality is that it is unlikely to happen for most kids. At least not right away. Start with tiny goals and celebrate when you and your child have accomplished them.

❷ **Set SMART mini-goals.** SMART stands for specific, measurable, attainable, relevant, and time bound. In other words, try to avoid goals like, "I want my kids to eat better"; instead, aim for a goal like, "For 5 out of the next 7 days, I will make one meal for the whole family." This is specific—you know exactly what you need to do. You can measure if you've done it or not. It is doable. It is an important step in undoing picky. And you've put a date on it—1 week. Additionally, it is very process centered—that is, you have total control over whether you achieve it. This is different than an outcome-centered goal such as "My kids will *eat the dinner* I make for them at least 5 out of 7 of the next days." You don't really have control over that. But by making the family meals, you increase the odds the kids will eat them.

❸ **Invest in the process.** The best way to undo picky eating is to invest in the process rather than outcome. Changing any behavior takes a lot of time and patience. This is the rule rather than exception when it comes to training a child's taste buds to accept a wide variety of foods, especially if this selective eating is particularly pronounced or long-standing. The Picky Eater Project process works, but for some kids it will take a much longer time than others. Reward yourself along the way for doing your part, which is ultimately all you can control.

❹ **Automate a plan.** Come up with a well-defined plan for how you would like to go about the daily task of feeding your children, and then put that plan on autopilot. Stick with it day in and day out, to the extent you can. We've put together of an example of what a plan might look like in Box 7.1.

❺ **Thrive on routine.** Kids thrive on routine, and you can, too. Identify and resist outside pressures that will break the family eating and mealtime routine, such as sports schedules and other activities, late nights at work, vacations, and visitors. That's not to say to avoid these activities altogether or be completely inflexible; rather, be proactive in trying to protect your family routines. This will not only help your once-picky eaters come around but also provide a degree of reliability, calm, and sense of ritual to your family. These are the experiences the kids will remember as they grow up.

❻ **Plan for problems.** A pros and cons chart doesn't work so well when you are trying to decide whether to make a change (we often tend to talk ourselves out of changing), but it sure does come in handy when in you're in the midst of it. Try to think of as many ways the plan could fail as you can. Then, come up with a solution of what you will do if each of those events were to happen (see a sample of this in Table 7.1).

Box 7.1. The Picky Eater Project Plan

Every family will have its own plan, but we would like to offer a sample one to help you automate yours. Routine is the essence of life, and kids thrive particularly well on it. Establish your routine, and much of the rest will fall into place.

Picky Eater Project Sample Plan

Sundays. Plan meals for the week. Purchase all needed groceries. Write out the meal plan. Make sure most dinners take no more than 30–45 minutes to prepare (caveat: when you include children, it will take time). When possible, prep in advance and freeze.

Sunday–Thursday Evenings. Pack lunches and snacks. Build lunches keeping a balanced plate/MyPlate in mind. Include a fruit, a vegetable, or both at each lunch and with each snack.

Monday–Friday. Kids sit down for breakfast by 7:30 am before leaving for school. Breakfast always includes at least one fruit.

After school/after practice snack is at least 2 hours before dinner. Otherwise, no snack needed. Snack includes at least a fruit, a vegetable, or both most of the time.

Spend 30–45 minutes preparing dinner. Involve your kids as often as possible.

Around 6:30 pm, eat dinner together as a family. Aim to eat at home at least 5 nights per week. Include a protein, whole grain, fruit, and vegetable at each dinner. Make sure your kids do their part in cleaning up.

Desserts on Wednesdays and Saturdays (more or less frequently depending on your preferences). By planning when you will have dessert, the kids will know when to expect it and will be less likely to ask or plead for it on other days.

While life will happen and it won't always be possible to stick to the plan, by simply having one, family meals will become more enjoyable and your kids will start to venture outside of their comfortable, go-to foods to try something new and eventually come around to liking it.

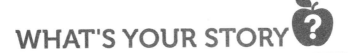

WHAT'S YOUR STORY

What have been some of the greatest challenges you've faced during your Picky Eater Project? What might be some ways to overcome these challenges in the future?

Table 7.1. Overcoming Obstacles

Part of any behavioral change is figuring out how to deal with obstacles and relapses and still get back on track. The table below lists possible challenges that might arise when participating in the Picky Eater Project and possible solutions to overcome them.

What Could Go Wrong	What to Do About It
Child who refuses to eat	Try to be OK with a child who refuses to eat a meal. Many times this happens because your child is simply not hungry (usually late afternoon snacks are the culprit). Resist temptation to cater to pickiness. Instead, remind your child that what is served is dinner and no other food will be available later. Encourage your child to listen to her signs of hunger and fullness and if she isn't hungry; it is OK to not eat. Do NOT make a separate meal. If this is an ongoing pattern and you are genuinely concerned your child is not eating enough to grow, check in with your child's pediatrician to assess growth, weight, and potential underlying issue. See Chapter 8 for further discussion of health concerns associated with severe picky eating.
Partner/spouse/ grandparent or some other very important person who refuses to go along with the project/plan	Try to get this person on board. If that fails, readdress in 1 month. In the meantime, do everything you can to follow rules of "picky-free parenting." Refer back to Chapter 1 discussion on the rules of picky-free parenting. See page 13 for review.
Child with friends who impede progress	Reinforce rules that occur in your house to support more adventurous eating. Encourage or arrange for your child to spend more time with other friends who are more adventurous. Assess how much of a negative effect it is really having. (If it is a big effect, come up with a game plan to address it such as inviting your child's friend to your house for meal or snack times, arranging playdates that may not involve food, or taking very small steps to help your child's friend come around to liking healthier foods, too.)
Short on time	Plan meals ahead on the weekends. If there is a need to eat prepackaged foods or dine out, choose meals with all the main food groups (whole grain, protein, vegetable, and fruit). Avoid children's menus as a general rule as most of the time they cater to children's preferences for foods such as chicken fingers, macaroni and cheese, cheese pizza, and hot dogs and are loaded with calories, sugar, and salt.

Table 7.1 *(cont)*

What Could Go Wrong	What to Do About It
Short on money	Buy in bulk and plan meals in advance to use different variations of similar ingredients. Seek out coupons and specials. Choose frozen and canned produce when more economical than fresh. Assess eligibility for nutrition support programs such as SNAP (Supplemental Nutrition Assistance Program) and WIC (Women, Infants, and Children).
Short on energy or patience	Start with one small change to move closer to the overall goal and follow it consistently. Recognize when energy or patience is wearing thin, pause, and remind yourself of your one small goal.
Multiple schedules to coordinate	Create a weekly family planner. Carve out as many days as possible for family dinners. We suggest a minimum of 3, with a goal of many more than that. Adjust schedules and activities to make this a priority.
Multiple picky eaters to engage	Implement a one-family, one-meal policy. Incorporate foods that all will like but try not to worry if they don't.
Not a fan of cooking	Choose very simple meals and try to motivate yourself to cook with your kids at least once per week. Do this with the goal of gradually increasing your kids' responsibilities in the kitchen so that eventually one or more of them may be ready to take over at least parts of meal preparation. Ask yourself if anything might help you like cooking more. If yes, pursue that.
Incompatible parenting style	If your natural inclination is to pressure your kids to clean their plates, or jump up to cater to a child's gripes, you may find that the picky-free parenting approach is very difficult. Ask yourself what your major goal is from this project and assess if it is something that requires a change in parenting approach to achieve. If so, start with very small, specific goals to train yourself to respond in a way that may not feel natural.
Forgot about the plan, and regressed into the old ways	Recognize the minor lapse and recommit. Start the Picky Eater Project over, or jump in where you left off. Remind yourself that life happens and get back on the plan.
Concerned about food waste	Introduce new foods in small portions. Serve yourself smaller portions in anticipation of eating kids' leftovers. Freeze leftovers for another day or use leftover ingredients to make a twist on the same meal or pack leftovers in lunches for school or work. Compost foods scraps.

❼ Rally support. Let your family and friends know you are on a mission to take back mealtimes. Offer updates and ask them to hold you accountable to not become stressed when your child refuses a new food or refuses to eat one day. Engage with your social networks to share your stories, troubleshoot problems, and find support.

❽ Involve your kids every step of the way. Remember, the changes you are trying to make will occur on a family level. Involve your kids at every turn—starting from the very beginning with the goal-setting session. Take their preferences into consideration and work together to achieve your shared goal. If they aren't ready to begin this change, work with them to come around, using some of the strategies we discuss in Chapter 6, such as positive modeling and peer influence, on pages 167 through 169. Make strides with them instead of forcing something upon them. Try to be OK with it if that means taking baby steps when you were hoping to leap.

❾ Commit. Post your 10 rules of "picky-free parenting" in a visible place to serve as a reminder of your plan, as well as a reminder to the family that you have committed to put a stop to mealtime battles for good.

❿ Celebrate. Too often we experience small and large degrees of success and never come around to celebrating. Celebrate the small successes. You'll get an instant surge of energy and recharge to keep up with your plan.

YOUR PICKY EATER PROJECT

Post-Picky Eater Project: Making It Stick-y

Project To-dos Checklist

☐ Perform a final check-in with the goals you established in week 1. How far have you come? How much is left to be done? Use this information to help establish goals for round 2.

☐ Sketch out your own weekly feeding plan. Each week do everything you can to stick with your plan.

☐ As outlined in Table 7.1 on page 194, create a list of worst-case scenarios, of what can go wrong, as you try to keep up the changes you've made over the past 6 weeks. For each one, write down what you will do to overcome that challenge, if it occurs.

☐ Tally any major challenges or relapses that have occurred so far. How did you handle them?

Project Check-in

❶ What was your Family Mealtime Mission Statement you outlined in week 1?

❷ What was your vision of what success would look like by the end of this project?

❸ On a scale of 1 to 10 (1 being no change; 10 being complete transformation), how far did you come with your Picky Eater Project? Why did you pick the number you picked? What remains to be done?

❹ On a scale of 1 to 10 (1 being very peaceful; 10 being all-out war), how would you rate the enjoyableness of your mealtimes prior to beginning the Picky Eater Project? What would you rank it now? What changed?

❺ On a scale of 1 to 10 (1 being not at all; 10 being strictly), how well did you follow your "picky-free parenting" rules over the course of the 6 weeks? What was difficult? What was easy?

❻ What new foods did your children try over the course of the 6 weeks?

❼ Who has been the most supportive of this project? Who has been the least supportive? How did the support (or lack thereof) affect your Picky Eater Project?

❽ What experience sticks out the most from your Picky Eater Project?

❾ What change from the past 6 weeks are you most proud of?

The formal portion of the Picky Eater Project is complete, but the changes and opportunities will continue. What will be your next goal to help you achieve your vision of what success will look like in 6 months? Consider the tips in this chapter to help you answer this question. But while motivation and a defined period of time for a project can help spark some pretty significant changes, eventually life catches up. Any behavioral change is difficult to maintain and roadblocks may come up along the way. Keeping it going for the long haul is a real challenge—at first. But day by day as new habits set in, you will find that the lifestyle changes you have made not only help relieve the stress of picky eating but, more important, set the stage for happier, healthier family mealtimes.

CHAPTER 8

Troubleshooting

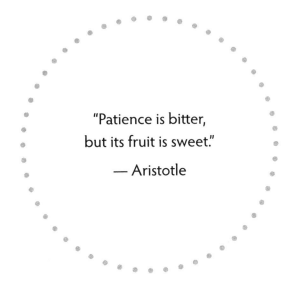

"Patience is bitter,
but its fruit is sweet."

— Aristotle

Mission
Improve eating habits of even the most severe picky eaters.

Strategy
Identify the underlying cause of severe picky eating and take
steps to address it.

Measurement
Number of signs of progress, no matter how small.

As was the case for Brooke and Hunter, in most cases picky eating is a normal developmental stage that in some cases can linger too long. It is very responsive to the strategies described in the 6 weeks of the Picky Eater Project. However, sometimes picky eating can become severe, affecting a child's growth and acting as an impediment to everyday functioning for the child and family. In these cases, severe picky eating is often a manifestation of a physical or mental health condition in the child or a sign of an alarming incompatibility in a child's personality and parent feeding style. When this occurs, it is important to be able to recognize the signals (see Health Alert: Red Flags section on page 202), discuss them with your child's pediatrician, and implement an individualized plan to help your child and your family thrive. While the process may take longer for children with severe picky eating, in most cases, patient implementation of a variation of the Picky Eater Project along with help from a team of health professionals such as a pediatrician, occupational therapist, and pediatric psychologist can have a significant positive effect.

So how do you know what is picky eating that is very responsive to interventions, such as the Picky Eater Project, versus *severe* picky eating, which may be more resistant to change, is life altering, and is potentially a sign of a co-occurring or an underlying health concern?

Having a game plan to stick to such as the Picky Eater Project is a good start. If you've seen some notable progress and found that your child (and the rest of the family) is enjoying mealtimes a little bit more and overall thriving, chances are good that the picky eating will fade. In this case especially, as Aristotle noted more than 2,000 years ago, "patience is bitter, but its fruit is sweet." However, if you complete the project and you've seen no change, or your child demonstrates any of the red flags described next, it is important to address your concerns with your child's pediatrician and assess whether further evaluation or intervention is needed, or if the best course of action may be repeating the Picky Eater Project.

Health Alert: Red Flags

Red flags can be divided into 2 types, though there is some overlap. The first are red flags that may indicate an underlying health problem. These include

- Failure to grow or gain weight

- Difficulty chewing or swallowing

- Passage of food or liquids into the lungs (aspiration)

- Pain or apparent pain with feeding

- Vomiting or diarrhea associated with eating

- Developmental delays

- Some lung or heart problems, such as cystic fibrosis or congenital heart disease

The second are red flags that may indicate an underlying mental health or social problem. These include

- Extreme selectivity to the point of having only a handful of tolerable foods

- Forceful feeding by a caregiver

- Sudden rejection of food after a choking or an otherwise traumatic event

- Anticipatory gagging

- Failure to grow or gain weight

- Refusal to eat or fear of fat

- Excessive weight loss or insistence on maintaining a very low body weight

- Compensatory behaviors such as vomiting or excessive exercise after eating

If a child shows signs of any of the above red flags, a prompt medical evaluation is needed.

Identifying Possible Health Conditions

Health problems that can trigger or present with severe picky eating can generally be divided into 3 categories: *limited appetite, selective intake,* and *fear of feeding.* The conditions that fit under each of these categories as well as what to do about them are detailed in Table 8.1. In some cases an underlying medical or mental health cause of the severe pickiness is not identified. In that situation, some kids may meet the criteria for a feeding disorder called avoidant/restrictive food intake disorder (ARFID).

Children with ARFID have such severe problems with eating that they are unable to consume enough calories or adequate nutrition through their diet. This can occur because of problems with food digestion, inability, or unwillingness to eat certain food colors or textures; eating very small portions; having no appetite; or being afraid to eat after a scare like choking or vomiting. Children with ARFID may not gain weight appropriately or may even lose weight.

Avoidant/restrictive food intake disorder should be diagnosed only after consultation with a qualified medical professional. The criteria for diagnosis include

- Persistent failure to meet appropriate nutrition or energy needs causing significant weight loss (or failure to gain weight), nutritional deficiency, dependence on tube feeding or oral nutrition supplements, interference with psychosocial functioning, or any combination of those.

- Disturbance cannot be explained by lack of available food or a culturally sanctioned practice.

- Disturbance does not occur exclusively during the course of another eating disorder (anorexia or bulimia nervosa) and there is no body image disturbance.

- The disturbance cannot be better explained by another medical or mental health condition.

Table 8.1. Possible Causes of Severe Picky Eating

This table is for informational purposes only. The information here is not intended to be construed as medical advice that would replace advice from your child's doctor. If you are concerned your child may have severe picky eating, consult your child's pediatrician.

Category	Description	Possible Interventions
Limited Appetite		
Misperceived parental response	Excessive parental concern despite normal growth	Practice responsive parenting strategies such as following the 10 rules of "picky-free parenting" (see Chapter 1 on page 13).
Energetic, active child	Child more interested in playing and talking than eating. Refuses to sit during meals, eats small amounts, and fails to gain weight. Oftentimes no underlying health problem. Can be associated with attention-deficit/hyperactivity disorder.	Practice responsive parenting. Teach your child to appreciate hunger and satiety cues. Implement a feeding schedule. **Plan** • Maintain a pleasant food environment. • Avoid distractions. • Limit mealtimes to 20 minutes. • Offer 4–6 meals/snacks per day. • Encourage self-feeding. Offer attention in response to positive behavior; withdraw attention for unacceptable behavior (see Table 8.2 on pages 207–210 for more information on this technique, known as "differential reinforcement"). If growth failure, supplementation may be needed.
Apathetic, withdrawn child	Disinterested in eating and environment May be associated with depression or eating disorder such as anorexia nervosa	Provide adequate nutrition and supportive meal environment. Seek pediatrician advice. May need additional outside help as often this is associated with a poor child-parent attachment or mental health concerns.
Underlying health condition	Organic disease as cause for limited appetite, often gastrointestinal, cardiovascular, neurologic, or metabolic	Seek pediatrician advice.

Table 8.1 *(cont)*

Category	Description	Possible Interventions
Selective Intake		
Misperception	Neophobia misunderstood	Repeated exposure to foods increases acceptability (see Table 8.2).
Mild selectivity	Limited tolerable foods; not responsive to repeated exposures	Consistently apply responsive parenting strategies despite urge to engage in coercive or indulgent practices, which make the problems worse.
Highly selective	Limit diet to 10–15 foods. Tend to have sensory food aversions, refusing whole categories of foods related to taste, texture, smell, temperatures, or appearance. Can affect oral motor skills.	Food bridges, fading, and shaping may be effective (see Table 8.2).
Underlying health condition	Sensitive responses to food or delayed oral motor skills. Gags in anticipation of food touching mouth. Associated conditions include • Developmental delays resulting from neurologic, mitochondrial, and chromosomal disorders • Sensory integration disorder	Resistant to standard treatments Occupational therapy May include sensory integration, including tactile exposure on skin and then oral motor desensitization, shaping, and fading (See Table 8.2.)

Table 8.1 *(cont)*

Category	Description	Possible Interventions
Fear of Feeding		
Misperception	Babies with excessive crying or who resist bottle or breast. Most often crying for other reasons, such as colic or the inability to self soothe.	Patient parenting. Work with pediatrician to attempt to identify underlying cause. Soothing measures (eg, swaddle, suck, sway).
Event related	Fear after a single event like choking or subject to painful procedures or parental force feeding	Parental reassurance Therapy
Underlying medical condition	Fear of a painful experience resulting from eating Associated conditions include • Gastroparesis • Disordered small bowel motility • Food allergies • Esophagitis • Anxiety disorder	Treatment of underlying disorder. Possible evaluation by allergist if there is concern for food allergies. Signs of a food allergy may include vomiting or stomach cramps, dizziness, coughing or wheezing, shortness of breath, tongue swelling, or in severe cases anaphylaxis. The most common culprits are eggs, milk, peanuts, tree nuts, fish, shellfish, wheat, and soy. If any of these symptoms occur after eating a food, discuss with your child's pediatrician. Call 9-1-1 for severe symptoms. Mental health referral for therapy to reduce anxiety associated with feeding and eating. Medication and supplementation may be necessary.

Table 8.2. Feeding Strategies That May Help Some Children With Severe Picky Eating
The following strategies may help encourage a child who is severely picky to try a new food. For many children with severe picky eating, these strategies may be most successful with the help of a feeding specialist, such as an occupational therapist or pediatric psychologist.

Strategy	Description	Examples	Recipe
Bridging	Introduce new foods that are very similar in taste or texture to a food the child already likes.	Pumpkin pie bridges to sweet potato pie, which bridges to mashed sweet potatoes, which bridges to mashed butternut squash, which bridges to mashed carrots, which bridges to roasted carrots, which bridges to raw carrots. **Initially preferred food** Pumpkin. **New foods** Sweet potatoes, butternut squash, carrots.	Sweet Potato Bar *(with variations)* (See Chapter 5, page 159.)

Table 8.2 *(cont)*

Strategy	Description	Examples	Recipe
Fading	Subtle transition from preferred food or texture to a new food or texture. **Simultaneous presentation** A small amount of new or non-preferred food is mixed with a preferred food. Initially the new food is indiscernible but then gradually the amount is increased. **Prompt fading** Initially child practices picking up food and then moves food toward mouth, then into mouth. **Size fading** Start with very small bite. Touch lip, touch tongue, place in mouth, chew and spit, and then chew and swallow. Gradually increase bite size. **Texture fading** Start with preferred texture, such as pureed food. Then fade to finely chopped, to chopped, and to bite-sized.	Start with a fruit smoothie. Add small amount of spinach or kale for a "green smoothie" that tastes mostly the same but color has changed. Further increase spinach or kale so the taste is somewhat recognizable. **Initially preferred food** Fruit smoothie. **New food** Spinach or kale paired with sweet taste in green smoothie.	Green Monster Smoothie (See page 215.)

Table 8.2 (cont)

Strategy	Description	Examples	Recipe
Shaping	Behavior is broken down into small steps. Each step is positively reinforced with praise, attention, or other reward.	Prepare a food or meal that has a delicious smell. Invite the child to help prepare the food, or at least smell it. Place the food on the child's plate. Allow child time to examine the food. Prompt but do not force or require the child to lick the food. If the child does, prompt but do not force to taste a small bite. If the child does, prompt but do not force to take a bigger bite.	Oatmeal Cookies (See page 216.)
Pairing	Introduce a new food alongside a food a child already likes.	Pair bitter tastes with generally more preferred sweet or salty tastes (eg, broccoli with cheese).	Broccoli Cheddar Soup (See page 218.)
Repeated exposure	Offer the child the same food repeatedly over time.	Introduce one new food at a time. Offer a small amount at the beginning of the meal. If refused, offer again in a similar or new way in 3–5 days.	Tomatoes—Any Way You Want Them (See page 220.)
Motivation to eat	Children will be most open to eating a new food if they are hungry.	Schedule meals and limit snacks to ensure a child is hungry at the time of a new food introduction. Introduce foods you most want child to eat when the child is the hungriest.	The Salad (See Chapter 3, page 89.)

Table 8.2 *(cont)*

Strategy	Description	Examples	Recipe
Social modeling	Child witnesses another person the child likes or admires eating the food, such as a sibling, friend, or parent.	Parent models eating a variety of foods at meal-times. Parent never asks child to eat something the child will not eat.	Make-it-your-way meals such as Sandwich Mix and Match, The Salad, Fajitas, and Fish Tacos (See pages 83, 89, 155, and 157, respectively.)
Differential reinforcement	Provide positive attention and reward for desired behaviors and ignore undesired behaviors.	Meal "time out" in which praise and positive attention is given when child makes progress in feeding and when child is disruptive or not adherent, attention is withdrawn.	Any meal

Some children may not show the red flags but be at risk for severe picky eating nonetheless. Researchers have found that there is a higher risk for severe picky eating with prolonged, disruptive, or stressful mealtimes; little encouragement or opportunity for independent feeding; late-night eating in toddlers; use of distraction to encourage a child to eat more; prolonged breast or bottle-feeding; and failure to advance textures. Developmental periods when risk of developing these features is high include transition periods such as moving from breast to bottle or cup, solid food introduction, and self-feeding.

First Steps in Battling Picky Eating Habits

The first step for any child who exhibits picky eating but not any of the red flags previously discussed is a close assessment of the family feeding environment. Countless studies have supported that an "authoritative"/"responsive"/"picky-free parenting" approach is most effective for raising healthy eaters. This is the approach described in week 1 and throughout the book: parents create structure and set the stage for healthy and more adventurous eating, but children are given some choices and autonomy. If that is not the natural parenting approach, the family may benefit from a trial period in which caregivers attempt to adopt a more responsive parent feeding approach instead of the other styles such as neglectful (little to no attention is paid to feeding at all); authoritarian/controlling, in which children are pressured or forced to eat foods; and permissive/indulgent, in which parents beg and plead for a child to eat and prepare special foods and meals. While the challenge of severe picky eating can feel overwhelming and sometimes even insurmountable, with patience and help, a change in parent feeding style can often lead to substantial improvements in the foods a child will eat.

You can get a good sense of your style by considering the following questions:

- How anxious are you about your child's eating?

- How would you describe what happens during mealtime?

- What do you do when your child won't eat?

Answers to these questions along with the Child Feeding Questionnaire in week 1 of the Picky Eater Project (see Chapter 1, Tables 1.1–1.4, on pages 9–11) will help in assessing your feeding style.

Ultimately, every child with picky eating is different and benefits from an individualized plan in partnership with a pediatrician and other health professionals.

YOUR PICKY EATER PROJECT

Troubleshooting

Project To-dos Checklist

☐ Identify if your child shows any red flags that could indicate an underlying physical or mental health problem. If your child does, discuss this with your child's pediatrician.

☐ Whether or not your child shows red flags, discuss your concerns with your child's pediatrician and get a better sense if referral to an occupational therapist, a pediatric psychologist, a registered dietitian, or another health professional may be helpful. Be sure to get a sense of how well your child is growing to better understand how much the picky eating may be affecting your child's nutritional status.

☐ If you haven't already, complete the Picky Eater Project. It is OK to take longer than 1 week for each area of focus, if needed. Pay special attention to your parenting approach, and aim to adopt an "authoritative"/"responsive"/"picky-free parenting" style as possible.

Project Check-in: "Slow Is Smooth, and Smooth Is Fast"

❶ How confident do you feel you will be able to affect your child's picky eating preferences? What would it take to feel more confident?

❷ How might the information from this chapter influence your approach with your child when it comes to mealtimes and feeding practices?

❸ What one thing do you do plan to do differently? How will you know if it was successful?

❹ Who else might you consider engaging to help you address your child's severe picky eating (eg, pediatrician, other health professionals, family member, friend)?

❺ How much time, energy, and resources are you willing to invest in helping your child overcome picky eating? How will you implement your plan? How will you measure your progress?

Note: Much of the information in this chapter is derived from the following 2 excellent articles on severe picky eating:

- Kerzner B, Milano K, MacLean WC, Berall G, Stuart S, Chatoor I. A practical approach to classifying and managing feeding difficulties. *Pediatrics.* 2015;135(2):344–353
- Zucker N, Copeland W, Franz L, et al. Psychological and psychosocial impairment in preschoolers with selective eating. *Pediatrics.* 2015;136(3):e582–e590

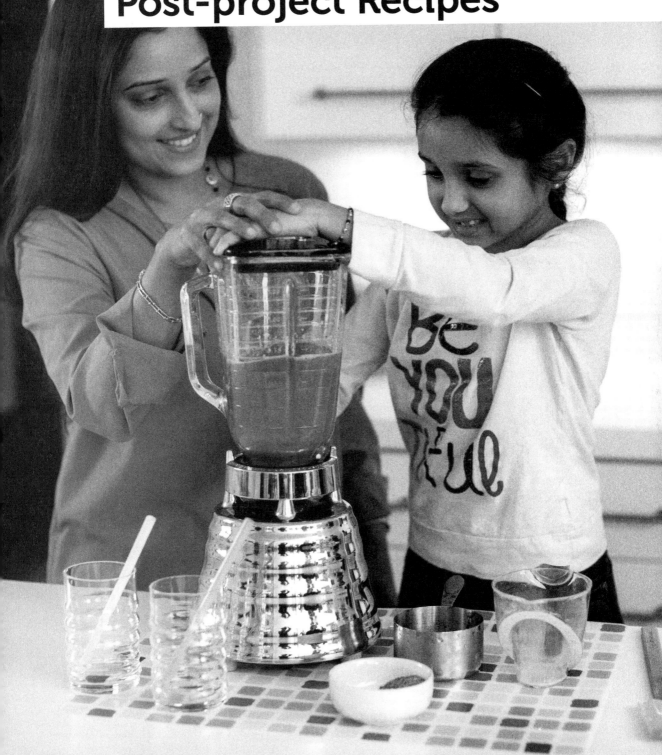

Post-project Recipes

Green Monster Smoothie

Hands-on time: 15 minutes
Total time: 15 minutes
Makes: four ¾-cup servings

Add spinach or kale to your smoothie and it looks like something that oozed out of a swamp—but it tastes great and has monster nutrition. Kids will love the name and green color!

Kitchen Gear

Sharp knife

Cutting board

Measuring cup

Measuring spoons

Blender

Ingredients

2 cups chopped kale leaves

1 overripe banana, sliced (If you plan ahead, freeze the peeled banana before making the smoothie.)

1 apple, cored and chopped

1 cup frozen blueberries

1 cup plain yogurt

½ cup orange juice

2 tablespoons toasted almonds or walnuts (if you like)

Instructions

1. Combine the kale, banana, apple, blueberries, yogurt, orange juice, and almonds or walnuts (if you like) in the blender. Put the top on tightly.

2. Turn the blender to medium and blend until the mixture is very smooth.

3. Serve right away, or store in a thermos or fridge up to 4 hours.

Personalize It

Add or swap any of the ingredients with other fruits and vegetables, like kiwi, avocado, or spinach.

Kids in the Kitchen

- Let your child measure and add all the ingredients to the blender.

- Toast your own almonds or walnuts.

- Let your child tear the kale using clean hands.

Oatmeal Cookies

Hands-on time: 20 minutes
Total time: 35 to 80 minutes, depending on how many batches you bake
Makes: 5 to 6 dozen

Kitchen Gear

Measuring cup

Measuring spoons

Large mixing bowl

Rubber spatula

Spoon

Baking sheet

Pot holder

Large plate

Ingredients

2 sticks unsalted butter, at room temperature

½ cup white sugar

1 cup light brown sugar

2 large eggs, at room temperature

1 tablespoon vanilla extract

2 cups quick-cooking or old-fashioned rolled oats

1 cup all-purpose flour

½ cup whole-wheat flour

1 teaspoon baking soda

1 teaspoon kosher salt

Instructions

1. Turn the oven on and set it to 325 degrees Fahrenheit.

2. Combine the butter, white sugar, and brown sugar in a bowl and mix until smooth and creamy.

3. Add the eggs and vanilla extract and mix well.

4. Scrape down the sides of the bowl; add the oats, flour, baking soda, and salt; and beat until everything is mixed well. (You can cover and refrigerate the dough up to 1 week.)

5. To form the cookies, break off small pieces of dough and roll into heaping teaspoon-sized balls and place them about 2 inches apart on a baking sheet. Using your palm, gently press each ball down to flatten slightly.

6. Carefully put the baking sheet in the oven and bake until the cookies begin to brown at the edges, 12 to 15 minutes. Cool on the baking sheet. Transfer to a plate and repeat with the remaining dough.

Personalize It

Add any of the following ingredients to your cookies:

- Walnuts
- Chocolate chips
- White chocolate chips
- Dried cranberries
- Unsweetened cocoa powder

Kids in the Kitchen

- Let your child measure and add each ingredient to the mixture.
- Share the task of rolling the dough into balls and flattening them on the baking sheet.

Broccoli Cheddar Soup

Hands-on time: 15 minutes
Total time: 45 minutes
Makes: 6 to 8 servings

Broccoli is rarely on the list of kids' top foods and this soup may change all that. Since broccoli is so often overcooked (code for stinky and mushy), the key is to cook it briefly.

Kitchen Gear

Measuring spoons

Sharp knife

Cutting board

Measuring cup

Grater

Large heavy-bottomed pot

Pot holder

Blender or food processor

Slotted spoon

Clean dish towel

Ingredients

1 tablespoon canola, vegetable, or olive oil or unsalted butter

1 large onion, coarsely chopped or thinly sliced

1 carrot, scrubbed or peeled, and chopped

1 celery stalk, sliced

1 garlic clove, peeled, and minced or chopped

1 head broccoli, divided into stalks and florets

8 cups low-sodium chicken or vegetable broth

¼ cup brown rice or 1 potato, scrubbed and cubed (if you like)

1 cup grated cheddar cheese

Instructions

1. Place the pot on the stove and turn the heat to medium. When it is hot, carefully add the oil.

2. Add the onion, carrot, celery, garlic, and broccoli *stalks* and cook until tender, 10 to 15 minutes.

3. Add the chicken broth and rice or potato; raise the heat to high and bring to a boil.

4. Lower the heat to low, add the broccoli *florets,* and cook uncovered until the broccoli is tender and bright green, about 15 minutes.

5. Transfer to a blender or food processor, add the cheese, and blend in batches until smooth.

6. Serve right away or cover and refrigerate up to 3 days.

Personalize It

- Add other vegetables to your soup, like corn, squash, or mushrooms.

- Substitute fontina cheese for the cheddar.

- Substitute plain yogurt for the cheddar cheese.

- Add ¼ cup chopped fresh basil when you blend the soup.

Kids in the Kitchen

- Let your child add all the ingredients to the pot and cook.

- Count how many vegetables are being used in this recipe.

- Taste test the soup before serving: Does it need more broth? Does it need a squeeze of lemon juice? Does it need a grinding of black pepper?

Tomatoes—Any Way You Want Them

Hands-on time: 15 minutes
Total time: 45 minutes
Makes: 6 to 8 servings

Instructions

Raw with dip or a sprinkle of salt. Buy local and in season for the best taste.

Oven-Roasted Tomatoes

Hands-on time: 20 minutes
Total Time: 40 minutes
Makes: 4 to 6 servings

You can eat them hot or cold, alone, or paired with pasta or rice.

Kitchen Gear	**Ingredients**
Sharp knife	2 cups grape or cherry tomatoes (If using plum, cut in half and roast cut side down.)
Cutting board	
Measuring cup	2 garlic cloves, peeled and chopped
Measuring spoons	1 teaspoon olive oil
Mixing bowl	⅛ teaspoon dried thyme
Large baking sheet with sides	¼ teaspoon salt
Large spoon	⅛ teaspoon black pepper

Instructions

1. Turn the oven on and set it to 400 degrees Fahrenheit.

2. Put the tomatoes, garlic, olive oil, thyme, salt, and pepper in a bowl and mix well.

3. Pour the mixture onto the baking sheet, making sure the tomatoes are in a single layer. Transfer the baking sheet to the oven and bake until the tomatoes have shrunk and caramelized, about 45 minutes. Stir halfway through.

4. Serve right away or cover and refrigerate up to 2 days.

Personalize It

Add other chopped vegetables to roast!

- Onion
- Bell pepper
- Squash
- Zucchini

Kids in the Kitchen

- Purchase different types of tomatoes and do a taste test before and after roasting.
- Let your child mix the ingredients and pour it on the pan.

World's Quickest Tomato Sauce

Hands-on time: 20 minutes
Total time: 35 minutes
Makes: 4 to 6 servings

This easy, all-purpose tomato sauce can be used on any shape pasta, polenta, rice, quinoa, or barley.

Tip: When this sauce is completely cooled, pour it in an ice cube tray. When the sauce has frozen, put the cubes in a freezer bag for up to 2 months.

Kitchen Gear	Ingredients
Cutting board	2 teaspoons olive oil
Can opener	2 garlic cloves, peeled, and minced or chopped
Measuring spoons	1 tablespoon dried basil
Sharp knife	1 teaspoon dried oregano
Measuring cup	2 (28-ounce) cans diced tomatoes, including the liquid
Large skillet	2 tablespoons water
	¼ cup chopped fresh basil leaves
	Shaved or grated Parmesan cheese

Instructions

1. Place the skillet on the stove and turn the heat to medium-low. When the skillet is hot, carefully add the oil. Add the garlic, basil, and oregano and cook for 2 minutes.

2. Add the tomatoes and water and cook the tomato mixture until the color is closer to orange than red, about 15 minutes.

3. Sprinkle with Parmesan cheese and serve right away, or cool, cover, and refrigerate up to 3 days.

Index

Index